Managing your Mental He

MW00637652

Zoë J. Ayres

Managing your Mental Health during your PhD

A Survival Guide

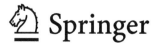 Springer

Written by
Zoë J. Ayres
Rugby, UK

Edited by
Petra Boynton

Illustrated by
Hana Ayoob

ISBN 978-3-031-14193-5   ISBN 978-3-031-14194-2   (eBook)
https://doi.org/10.1007/978-3-031-14194-2

This Springer imprint is published by the registered company Springer Nature Switzerland AG.
The registered company address is: Gewerbestrasse 11, 6330 Cham, Switzerland

This book is dedicated to all those who have lost their lives in the pursuit of higher education, all those who have felt alone in their struggles, and anyone who has ever thought they do not belong within the Ivory Tower.

Acknowledgements

After writing my PhD thesis, I thought I would never write a book again, but here we are. If nothing else I now have two very elegant door stops. Thank you to those of you who have believed in me when I have struggled to believe in myself. I am only here today due to a whole host of people who have enabled me to get to this moment, including family, friends, and the online #AcademicMentalHealth community who have given me encouragement every step of the way. Thank you to my husband Jonathan, who always supports me in my endeavours, even if he thinks I do far too much (and is probably right). Thank you to my parents for raising me to believe I can do anything. Fluffy, thanks for keeping me company and for deleting a whole page of this book I will never get back because of your love of head scritches and keyboards—I am sure it was not essential anyway. To my therapist Amy, thank you for working with me and enabling me to reconnect with who I am and what I want. You have honestly changed my life.

Thank you to Miriam Latuske for taking a chance on me on publishing this book, as well as a big thank you to Alina Cepraga, Sabine Schwarz, Srinivasan Manavalan, Martina Himberger, Jana Yagnavaragan, and the rest of the Springer team for helping me get to this point. To Dr Petra Boynton, thank you for reaching out to me (a complete stranger) and guiding me through the book publication process, for setting the foundations of speaking out and up for academic mental health long before I was on the scene, and agreeing to edit this book. Thank you for providing your expertise during the editing process. Hana Ayoob thanks for bearing with me and my terrible sketches and bringing my book cover and illustrations to life. A big thank you to Heloise Stevance, Hugh Kearns, and Maria Gardiner for permission to adapt their excellent graphics.

My anxiety is already getting the better of me, in that I might forget to thank someone, so I am sorry in advance if I do. You are appreciated.

I have had some amazing friends and colleagues who have stepped up to give me honest, critical feedback about my book prior to publication, or simply been there for me when I needed support, despite their busy schedules. Thank you to Juanita Limas, Mick Staniforth, Linda Corcoran, Heidi Gardner, Kevin Bolton, Daniel Ranson, Louise Burton, Natércia Rodrigues Lopes, Joe Ward, Ruth Patchett, Aya Abdalla, Christine Lockey, and the FOJ's (you know who you are!). Thank you to Nkasi Stoll, Amy Zile, Rachel Charlton-Dailey, Zofia Beck Anchondo, Rachel Cholerton, Marissa Edwards, and the whole Voices of Academia team, as well as anonymous contributors, for helping me with queries, questions, and perspectives when needed. Thank you to those of you that I have connected with from all over the world through social media that remind me why I do the work that I do and support me.

To my longest friend Stevie, I am super proud of you for choosing yourself over completing a PhD. I think this book is a step above our first book *The Ghost Story* from circa. ~1997 we wrote together, but the clip-art game is nowhere on a par. Thanks for always being there.

To my PhD supervisor Julie, thank you for supporting me through my PhD, including the bits I found particularly difficult to navigate, and championing me well beyond having left your lab. To Tania, Liz, Jenny, and Rob (and everyone else who I did my PhD with) thanks for making it all that bit more manageable, largely through laughter, memes, snacks, and the occasional shoulder to cry on.

Thank you to all of you who stepped forward and trusted me with your accounts of discrimination and bias—I do not think the book would pack as much punch without your contributions. Thank you for helping me drive for change and being living proof that anonymous stories help the tides of change as much as any other advocacy work.

Finally, I guess I should say thank you to past me. Thank you for persevering. Thank you for choosing to stay. I have never been more grateful or happier to be here. A lot can change in a few years. If this book helps even one person, it has been worth it. And even if it does not, I have realised somewhere down the road I am worth something anyway—that is more than enough for me.

Contents

About the Author

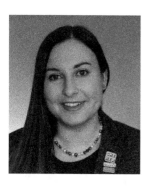

Zoë Ayres, (PhD) is an analytical scientist by profession, with a PhD in electrochemical sensor development. After spending several years as a postdoctoral researcher in academia post-PhD, she now works as an industry scientist. Additionally, Zoë is a mental health advocate, spurred on by experiencing mental illness herself during her PhD. Her advocacy work, drawing on lived experience, focuses on improving mental health in research settings, primarily focusing on PhD mental health. She raises awareness of the common issues PhD students face through various campaigns and initiatives, and can be found under the handle @zjayres on Twitter.

List of Figures

List of Tables

Part I

Defining the Problem

1

Introduction

Before We Start

Given the sensitivity of mental health, there may be topics that are difficult to read or may be triggering throughout this book. To help combat this, this guide has a detailed breakdown of the chapters and the content they cover at the start of the book. Additionally, trigger warnings (words or phrases that give an indication of the topics that will be discussed in the chapter that some readers may find distressing) are placed under each chapter title where intense topics are discussed, to help you navigate the book. I ask you to remember that for the sake of your mental health it is okay to take a step back from a topic, put this book down for a bit, or skip a chapter entirely.

When I started my PhD, I truly believed I was going to get my doctorate and change the world. I was filled with naïve optimism and a pinch of privilege thrown in for good measure. Before that point, nothing but my time and effort had stood in the way of my academic achievements. I can safely say that my PhD brought me down to earth—fast. I went from a person that was confident to someone constantly questioning their abilities, worrying for hours on end when my research simply was not working in the way I hoped it would. My research wasn't a success and from that I inferred neither was I.

Eventually, I ended up being diagnosed with clinical depression part way through my PhD. Again, I thought this was a reflection on me—that I was

---

(Trigger Warnings: suicidal ideation, depression)

Z. J. Ayres, *Managing your Mental Health during your PhD*,
https://doi.org/10.1007/978-3-031-14194-2_1

wholly inadequate and that I didn't have the resilience to survive in the academic environment. I felt so very alone. I thought that I was the only person experiencing mental illness, I was undeserving of my PhD position, and I would never be able to graduate. I was constantly bombarded with thoughts that I was not good enough, that I was a failure, and that I was letting everyone (including myself) down. But, unknowingly to myself at the time, it was the very skills that I had learnt by osmosis during my PhD program that were ultimately going to save my life. When I was at my lowest, at near breaking point, experiencing near daily suicidal ideation, I found myself at a crossroads. Unsure on how to proceed, I decided to do what any researcher might do: I started researching. I wanted to understand more about why I felt the way I did.

What I found shocked me. I learned that approximately 50% of PhD students experience mood disorders, such as anxiety and/or depression during their PhD [1]. Yes, you heard that right. 1 in 2 of our brightest minds. To put this in perspective this is about 6x higher than the general population [2]. I questioned why had I not heard about this endemic that was inherent within the PhD population? Why had I not been taught more about the risk I might face during a PhD?

As I delved deeper, I looked for books, papers, articles and resources talking about PhD mental health and found few. No PhD specific mental health support was offered to me at my institution. In fact, back then, I couldn't find tailored PhD mental health support at many institutions around the world.[1]

Over the years I've reflected on why this gap exists, and I have come to several conclusions. First, universities focus so heavily on undergraduate mental health that postgraduate mental health often falls by the wayside. This is understandable (to an extent) as undergrads typically make up the majority of the student populous. Combined with drastically underfunded, understaffed mental health support services, who are already stretched too thin, extending provision to postgraduate students seems a mammoth task [3]. What often ends up happening instead, is that undergraduate provision is garnered as appropriate for postgraduate students too, ultimately leading to mental health support feeling disingenuous. For example, the vast majority of PhD students are not having to deal with prolonged exam stress, so workshops or yoga sessions to "manage exam stress" are unlikely to feel useful to PhD students [4]. Further, despite working similar hours to academic staff, PhD students often do not qualify as "staff" at universities, meaning that they do not receive basic

---

[1] Thankfully this has really started to change over recent years, with more and more being published on PhD/graduate mental health and several universities realising the need to provide tailored support.

benefits like sick leave and employee mental health support [5]. And, in my experience, in the rare cases where PhD students are recognised as staff at their institutions, the mental health support for staff is not tailored for PhD students, and does not take into account the unique pressures of PhD study.

Second, is that mental health is nuanced and experiences from person to person are diverse. So much so, the onus for looking after one's mental health is often placed on the individual, despite our universities playing a huge role in feeding an often toxic research culture. Throughout my research, I have found that there are similar environmental challenges running through many individual experiences that impact mental health as a PhD student [6]. It is these common stress factors, that perhaps in isolation would be manageable, but combined together with the intensity of a PhD program, can lead to mental ill-health. This includes how we perceive ourselves and our achievements, for example, experiencing the impostor phenomenon, how we manage failure, and comparing ourselves with others, as well as institutional issues, such as experiencing poor supervision, systemic racism, and/or dealing with academic bullying [7]. All of which will be discussed throughout this guide.

Further, in my opinion, conversations around the systemic challenges that might be encountered are often not discussed before students embark on a PhD, as acknowledging there are issues means admitting there may be something that needs fixing in the first place. This silence is further exacerbated by PhD student mental ill-health being a concern at every institution around the world, as if the problem is everywhere, being among the first to step forward, acknowledge the issue, and work towards change, is a risk, requiring investment, resources, and prioritisation. Ignoring the issue, shifting blame, and relying on individual resilience, is often the perceived less costly approach (to our institutions).

And finally, perhaps the most prolific reason: there is still significant stigma attached to mental health. In the academic environment, many do not feel they can openly discuss their mental health for fear of losing future opportunities or being discriminated against [8]. Unfortunately, in many instances this is often true. *This must change.* It is only by talking about mental health that we can start to break the stigma that exists. We all have mental health— and to disregard it is to ignore a portion of us that enables us to do the world-leading research we joined academia to do.

This book aims to fill this gap that exists. We will explore the PhD experience like never before, focusing on your mental health, and all that may intersect with it during the PhD journey. This includes exploring how to improve your own wellbeing, from establishing a self-care strategy to seeking professional help. We will then delve deeper, focusing on parts of the academic journey that are outside of your control, that can be challenging.[2] As a "Survival Guide" this book by definition aims to explore beyond any personal responsibility to look after your mental health and delve into the systemic issues that exist within the academy that may impact wellbeing. To not discuss them would be to not describe what you need to "survive" through in the first place. There are of course plenty of amazing reasons we might want to embark on a PhD, such as loving to learn and wanting to make the world around us a better place (I suspect you would not be reading this book if you did not know what the positives of pursuing a PhD are). It is only natural that at the start of an exciting journey we focus on the positives and what we hope to get out of the process.[3] However, just like if you were to go on a long hike, setting off without a map and provisions could potentially be dangerous, the same is true of the PhD journey. It is this discussion that is so often missing when talking through the challenges of the academy. Thus in this book I hope to explore well beyond the typical, trite "eat well" conversation when it comes to mental health, and talk about the behind the scenes of doing a PhD that is so often missing. So yes, this book is going to be "self-help" for your PhD journey, but I hope it will be self-help with a difference.

Most of all, I want to say to you that, whether you are experiencing mental health concerns for the first time during your PhD, or have a long history with mental illness, you can succeed. A PhD is not for the exclusive few—there is space for us too.

1.1   A Comment on the Guide

An important disclaimer is that I'm no psychologist. Nor am I formally trained in mental health, and so this book is not intended to be a replacement for professional help, medical, legal advice, or otherwise. It is instead intended to be an insider guide on navigating your PhD, based on my own PhD journey and mental health advocacy work. A large portion of this book is experience-based for this reason, with reference to evidence-based statistics,

---

[2] Note: This book is not designed to discourage you from you endeavours. Far from it. Its purpose is to better prepare you for the personal challenges you may face navigating your PhD journey. As academics, we believe that with knowledge comes power: the same applies for PhD mental health. If you are aware of the challenges you may face and you are provided with coping strategies you can be better prepared and more likely to succeed.

[3] However, throughout, I aim to avoid "toxic positivity" which happens all too often, suggesting that everything about the PhD experience is fantastic, that we should be grateful for simply having a position, and nothing needs to be improved at an institutional level.

interventions, and resources that helped me, where appropriate. As I sit here writing, I know I will undoubtedly not capture everything out there. Because of this, there will be gaps in this book, literature I missed, perspectives I fail to cover, and amazing work I overlooked by accident. For me, this book has never been about creating an all-encompassing PhD mental health guide, where I come up with solutions for all challenges, but an opportunity to spark further discussion and change.

Some of the issues that I discuss in this book you may look at and think: "How would that affect my mental health?". The truth is that it is unlikely that every section will be relevant to you (and I sincerely hope they aren't). What I have learnt, however, is that with the PhD process, it is often the seemingly innocuous, small things, that in isolation would be manageable, when combined with others, that can take a huge toll on our mental health. This is why we will explore all the way from the perfectionism to discrimination and beyond.

Further, navigating mental illness while studying for a PhD can be tough. I want to acknowledge that I can give you all the advice in the world on how to manage your mental illness, but advice is not always helpful. This comes down to the fact that many of us are trying our best to be well, and the chances are that we have already tried a range of different options to manage our mental health. This guide in all likelihood will not offer a "quick fix" for you and solve the mental health struggles you are experiencing, but I do hope that it will make you realise you are not alone.

What I cannot do with this book is fix all the systemic issues within academia that you may encounter. Many are deeply ingrained, and certainly not possible to fix from the outside (although I will continue to actively campaign to make cross-sector changes). Any "tips and tricks" I can give you to navigate bullying or harassment, or experiencing microaggressions in the workplace, for example, run the risk of minimising how challenging it can be to be exposed to such serious issues. This is not my intention; I want to acknowledge that whilst throughout this book there is an emphasis on what you can do to empower yourself and seek help, focusing on the power you have, in order to address some of these issues fully, whole research culture reform is needed.

I also cannot cover every eventuality. The pressures that might contribute towards poor mental health and wellbeing are many, and as varied as the topics that we research. I have aimed to capture the key themes running through many mental health experiences during a PhD, but please note, if you do not find something covered, it does not mean your own experience is not valid. The PhD experience also varies vastly country to country. For example, there may be qualification for candidacy like in the US system, or vastly different lengths of a PhD program (for example in the EU, ~3.5 years is typical, whilst in the US PhD study is often much longer). To this end, I will refer to anyone studying for a PhD as a "PhD student" irrespective of how far into the process they are. Further the person that oversees a PhD Student may be referred to as a "Principal Investigator" in some countries, but for the purpose of this book I will use the name "PhD Supervisor", which is used more commonly in the UK. Some of these subtleties will be lost throughout this book, as this book is designed to provide advice and reassurance to PhD students globally.

This also highlights a much-needed disclosure from me, the author, at the start of this book. I studied for my PhD in the United Kingdom. I am a cis-gender, white woman, from a working-class background, who has depression and anxiety.[4] My own personal experience intersects with typical Science, Technology, Engineering and Technology (STEM) PhD study, but I have little experience of what doing a PhD is like outside this umbrella, for example, in the arts or humanities. Whilst I have broadened my perspectives, through my mental health advocacy work, as well as being a co-founder of the Voices of Academia blog (created to amplify the mental health stories of others), my experience will always be from my own lens, and tinged with my own biases.

I also want to take this opportunity to thank all the people that have shared their stories and struggles with me and enabled me to broaden my own understanding of the challenges that PhD students from all walks of life. You will find quotes throughout the book from a range of individuals, who are all PhD students unless explicitly stated otherwise. For each account, I have chosen to refer to individuals as simply "PhD Student 1", "PhD Student 2" etc. This is because some individuals intersect heavily with a range of different protected characteristics, and protecting their identity is paramount. Perhaps it is telling on academia that I have to do this. Those that contributed to this book represent experiences from a range of fields, from geography, to economics, to art history, to chemistry, from all genders, and from a range of countries across the world.

With a guide like this, there is always a trade-off between brevity, applicability of content, and the level of detail that is required to explore difficult topics. I hope that I have done each one of them justice, but I encourage you to seek out additional resources on topics covered here that resonate with you (please see the back of the book for information on how to access my online

---

[4] I am also mid-journey in seeking an Attention Deficit Hyperactivity Disorder (ADHD) diagnosis, which I believe has underpinned a large portion of my mental health journey (a story for another day).

PhD resource list). To this end, if there is one thing I truly hope to do with this book it is to empower you to seek out help for yourself locally, as relevant advice, accessibility, and availability of resources will also depend on your specific situation.

1.2 If You Are Studying for a PhD

I know that a PhD can be taxing, both in time and energy. For this reason, the book is broken down into short, digestible sub-sections, making it easier to stop and start reading the book when you can.

This guide focuses on four key sections. The first, "Defining the Problem Set" where we will look at the statistics behind PhD mental health, explore your understanding of mental illness, and drill down into why PhD mental health concerns are so high. The second can be simply summarised as "Mindset", looking at how you feel about yourself and how you can best support yourself through your PhD experience. I will cover a range of topics, from managing your research time, setting boundaries, and managing feeling like an impostor. I will also discuss a range of strategies to get you through your PhD program that you can work towards implementing **today**. The third part explores the common environmental stressors created by the existing research culture within academia that may impact your mental health during the PhD process. Many of these may not be directly in your control, and you may not have even noticed them, but I hope by acknowledging them as well as focusing on practical tips and tricks that you can do in order to navigate academia and stay well, I can empower you to succeed despite a research environment that may not be stacked in your favour. The fourth and final part of the book, explores seeking help for your mental health, including finding support groups, having difficult conversations with your supervisor, and putting yourself first.

Throughout each chapter I also provide some details of what institutions should and could be doing to make the PhD student experience better. I have included this because I want to challenge the notion that mental health is an individual issue. Responsibility for change relies heavily on our institutions recognising there is a problem and working towards a more equitable, welcoming research culture. I also include this to assist you as a PhD student, because although change so often should come top-down, often it is bottom-up, grassroots, student-led efforts that can make a difference when it comes to making change. In an ideal world you wouldn't have to advocate for yourself, but in this world that is far from that ideal, I give you a starting point to consider what you might lobby for.

I also want to emphasise that this book details some of the darker corners of academia—the bits we don't often openly talk about. It does not mean that everything detailed in this book will happen to you [9]. It is important to remember this.

1.3   If You Are a PhD Supervisor or PhD Course Coordinator

I want to start by saying that being a PhD Supervisor is a difficult, often thankless job, and the chances are if you are reading this book, you care deeply about the success and welfare of your PhD students already. On top of being a researcher, a leader, and a teacher, it is unreasonable to expect you to also act as a therapist or mental health provider to your PhD students as well. Quite frankly you are unlikely to be qualified to do so, let alone have the time to provide such support. However, you will likely be supporting a range of different PhD students through a challenging few years of their lives, and mental health concerns are going to feature along the way. I therefore ask you to think about how you can use your position to better improve PhD mental health support in two ways: (1) reflect on your own practices and the impact they could have (even inadvertently) and (2) consider how you might use your position of power to advocate for better mental health support for those that need it.

This book provides a starting point for you to understand some of the immense pressures students may be experiencing, enabling you to better support them through their PhD. I ask you to think about whether you know what resources are available to support someone if they came to you in distress, and find that information for a rainy day if you don't, as well as critically assess if the support that is available is fit for purpose. I also invite you to think about the role you might play in PhD student mental health, paying particular attention to Chap. 9.

Further, environments where mental health is never discussed can have huge impact on the wellbeing of your students. I encourage you to use this book as a starting point to have some of those difficult conversations. The "Advocating for Better" sections at the end of each chapter provide a good place to start.

1.4 If You Are a Concerned Friend or Family Member

You might be reading this book to better understand what a friend or family member is experiencing. Academia is nuanced with a hidden curriculum that can often impact PhD students heavily, but also, by proxy, family members and friends too. It can be incredibly difficult to put yourself in the shoes of your loved one who is embarking on a PhD. Academic terminology alone can result in difficulty communicating how someone is feeling to the "outside world". If you are reading this book, it is likely you have already noticed the signs of mental illness within your loved one and are looking for ways you can support them. I hope that this book can be used to better equip you to have much needed conversations. I also want to acknowledge that supporting someone with mental illness can be tough and to remind you that you yourself may also need support.

*   *   *

Finally, you may read this book, having already navigated a PhD and have not experienced any of the issues I explore. You may think that I am painting the academy in a particularly bleak light, and that I am providing only information on worst-case scenarios. I want to reiterate to you that survivor bias is very real, and just because you did not experience something that does not mean that it does not exist. Mental health struggles during PhD study are very real, and it is time for us to talk about it.

References

1. The Graduate Assembly (2014) Graduate student happiness & well-being report. University of California, Berkeley, CA
2. Evans TM, Bira L, Gastelum JB, Weiss LT, Vanderford NL (2018) Evidence for a mental health crisis in graduate education. Nat Biotechnol 36(3):282–284
3. Brown P (2016) The invisible problem? Improving students' mental health. Higher Education Policy Institute, Oxford, UK
4. Metcalfe J, Wilson S, Levecque K (2018) Exploring wellbeing and mental health and associated support services for postgraduate researchers. Vitae
5. Cornell B (2020) PhD life: the UK student experience. Higher Education Policy Institute, Oxford, UK

6. Mackie SA, Bates GW (2019) Contribution of the doctoral education environment to PhD candidates' mental health problems: a scoping review. High Educ Res Dev 38(3):565–578

7. Levecque K, Anseel F, De Beuckelaer A, Van der Heyden J, Gisle L (2017) Work organization and mental health problems in PhD students. Res Policy 46(4):868–879

8. Schueth A (2022) Reducing the stigma of academic mental health can save lives. Nat Rev Urol 19:129–130

9. Boynton P (2020) Being Well in Academia: Ways to Feel Stronger, Safer and More Connected. Routledge, Abingdon

2

Challenging Perceptions: What Is Mental Health Anyway?

I have noted that an assumption that is often made (at an institutional level and beyond) is that because we are highly educated individuals pursuing a PhD, we already know what mental health is and how to manage it. I am not going to make this assumption. I figure, if we are not taught about what mental health *is*, how on earth can we go on to manage it? Learning more about mental health from a holistic perspective definitely helped me, allowing me to actively work towards improving my own mental health management.

For our understanding it is important to differentiate between **mental health** and **mental illness**. Often used interchangeably there is a huge difference. Mental health is something we all have just like physical health and can be "good" or "bad" depending on our circumstances, fluctuating naturally. The World Health Organisation (WHO) defines mental health as "a state of wellbeing in which every individual realizes their own potential, can cope with the normal stresses of life, can work productively and fruitfully, and is able to make a contribution to their community" [1], and this is the definition I will use throughout this book. Being able to work "productively and fruitfully" and contribute to society underpins the PhD experience and is likely for many of us why we embark on a PhD in the first place. It is worth noting that this is idealised—no-one copes with stress perfectly every moment of every day or works productively all the time. Good mental health is achieving this state most of the time.

If our mental health is affected for a long period of time, it is possible to develop mental illness. It is something that some of us may never experience with approximately 1 in 10 in the world population having a mental illness [2]. Mental illness is described as "a range of mental health disorders that affect mood, thinking and behaviour" [3].

Not an exhaustive list, some mental illnesses that are present in the PhD population (as well as the general population) include eating disorders, such as Anorexia Nervosa and Binge Eating Disorder, Schizophrenia, Bipolar Disorder, Trichotillomania (hair pulling), Dermatillomania (skin picking), Post-Traumatic Stress Disorder (PTSD, including experiencing panic attacks), Obsessive Compulsive Disorder (OCD), Major Depressive Disorder (MDD, more commonly known as depression) and Generalised Anxiety Disorder (GAD) [4]. This means that providing holistic support to PhD students is a complex task. The good news is that mental illnesses are recognisable conditions, which means that with access to healthcare,[1] they can be professionally diagnosed, and a treatment plan can be put in place.

2.1   The Mental Health Continuum

There are a range of models to describe mental health and how mental illness intersect to assist with understanding. The one I find the most useful is the mental health continuum model discussed by Keyes (2002) [5]. A visual representation of the continuum, where mental health can be considered as a pressure dial, is illustrated in Fig. 2.1.

This model explores how mental health is something we all inherently have, just like physical health. On the continuum we can go from "flourishing" (being positive and healthy functioning) on the left to "languishing" (experiencing severe mental illness causing distress) on the right. Going from one to the other of these extremes can be sudden, but it can also be gradual, with many different stages along the way. From my experience, simplified for ease, the continuum can be broken down further into different stages as shown in Fig. 2.1. When we are in a good place with our mental health, matching the definition as described by the WHO, we sit on the left-hand side of the continuum. When our mental health is impacted, we move towards the right, as the pressure increases. Periods of high stress can move our position over to the right, with long-term exposure leading to distress and possibly triggering mental illness (where 1 in 2 PhD students find themselves) [6]. If left unchecked, mental health crisis can arise (illustrated by the dial being full,

---

[1] Access to healthcare is not always available and I want to acknowledge this. Inequity in healthcare can also contribute negatively to the PhD experience.

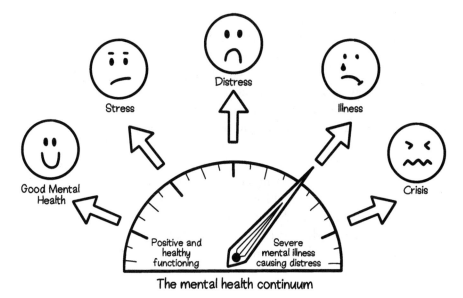

Fig. 2.1 A simplified Mental Health Continuum Model. Note: Whilst there are quantitative markings pictured on the dial, where we are on the dial at any one time is subjective, and dependent on our own experiences

resulting in the pressure building up so it becomes dangerous). Crisis can look different to different people, but may involve frequent thoughts of suicidal ideation and intentions to self-harm. In this situation immediate help is needed.[2]

Over the course of our lifetime our position on the mental health continuum may change; where exactly the needle on the dial sits at any one time depends on a combination of genetic factors as well as environmental factors [7]. Genetic factors can influence our susceptibility to mental illness [8]. This means that dependent on family history the needle may be intrinsically positioned more to the right than for someone with no family history of mental illness. This may mean result in being more predisposed to reaching a crisis point. Not all hope is lost, however. It is important to remember that even if we are predisposed to mental illness through genetic factors, this does not necessarily mean we will develop mental illness over the course of our lifetime. Further, although many of us may enter the academy with pre-existing mental illness, this does not mean we necessarily see worsening over time. With management, living with mental illness, and thriving, is absolutely attainable.

---

[2] If you find yourself here, please seek help. Options available to you are discussed in detail in Chap. 12.

Environmental factors also play a role in the pressure needle position [8]. Movement may be triggered by stressful events, such as the loss of a family member, hormonal changes, financial distress, juggling family life, physical illness, a global pandemic, or even embarking on a PhD program. Whilst many of these may be outside our control, fortunately, we can work to increase the capacity of the pressure dial and make it easier for us to manage our mental health. For example, access to the right medications, support structures, and accommodations can help us stay well. More on this in Chap. 4.

Systemic issues both inside the academy and out (discussed in detail in Chap. 8) such as racism, bullying and harassment, a poor supervisory relationship, financial concerns, ableism and more, also influence how we feel and the pressures we are under [9]. Of course, in these instances where the research culture we work in itself needs reform, the onus for change should not be on us, but until change is realised, we often have to draw on self-care and support for survival.

2.2   Barriers to Seeking Help

It is important to recognise that some of the common thoughts we might have when experiencing mental illness, can be internalised barriers that prevent us from seeking help. These can include common thoughts I had during my own mental health journey:

"I am not sick enough"—We tend to overestimate how long we must be struggling with our mental health before seeking help. In reality, if you are noticing a decline in your mental health away from your normal, even over short time periods, it may be time to go seek help from a medical professional.

"Others have it worse"—Comparing ourselves with others can be a dangerous game when it comes to our mental health. Everyone has different life experiences, different genetic factors and different environmental factors that influence their mental health. Just because someone else "has it worse" does not mean that you are undeserving of help. Struggling is relative to our own life experiences.[3]

"I'm doing everything right though"—We can have a fantastic self-care plan and be implementing it well to look after our mental health and think

---

[3] This was perhaps the most challenging barrier for me personally to face. I had a supportive partner, was surrounded by friends and family, and an excellent PhD Supervisor—what did I have to complain about? That is the thing with depression, our brains lie to us. it is also important to remember that suffering is not a competition.

that because it is not working that we are "unfixable". This isn't true. There is a range of medical, spiritual, and community-based support out there if you know where to look (discussed further in Chap. 12). It is also important to realise that self-care is not "one size fits all" and can be very different person to person.

"I should be grateful"—Everything might be fine in our lives (e.g., good friends, family, financial security) and yet we still struggle with our mental health. This can result in feelings of shame and guilt because we feel we should be grateful, and yet we cannot shake feeling low. It is important to remember that mental illness is exactly that—an illness. Even with the best support in place, it may take medical intervention and time to feel better.

"I don't deserve help"—Mental ill-health can often be combined with low self-worth. We can get caught up on the idea that those around us would be better off without us (not true). Everyone has value. Everyone is deserving of help to get better. This includes you.

It is also necessary to acknowledge that the barriers you might face, both internal and external, are dependent on our culture, ethnicity, religion, language, and more. This can make overcoming these barriers difficult (although difficult doesn't mean impossible).

2.3   Recognising the Signs

One of the biggest challenges when struggling with a mental illness is recognising and accepting that there is a problem in the first place. This is because we must face the fact that not only are we unwell, but that we are also *worthy of help*. How mental ill-health presents is different for different people. Here are some you may be experiencing [10, 11]:

- Anger, including channelling that anger internally towards yourself.
- Self-harming (including food restriction and/or binge eating).
- Feeling like you don't deserve to be where you are.
- Struggling to find joy, even in activities you used to enjoy.
- Intrusive, negative thoughts, including disaster spiralling.[4]
- Difficulty with motivation and/or concentration.

---

[4]To give you an example of disaster spiralling, for me personally, I might see that it is raining outside, think it might be more dangerous to drive in (which is true and important to be aware of), but then I might also think about all my loved ones and that they might get hurt in an accident because of it. Suddenly my thoughts have gone not from a to b, but from a to z in terms of hypothesised scenarios.

- Feeling that others will be better off without you.
- Experiencing suicidal thoughts.
- Finding it hard to feel anything at all (feeling emotionally numb).
- Feelings of tiredness/lethargy.
- Increased stimming.
- Feeling hopeless.
- Experiencing episodes of extreme hyperactivity (mania), followed by lows.

> **Stimming:** Repetitive body movements or noises, for self-stimulation, such as finger flicking, clapping, or rocking back and forth [12].

When struggling with your mental health it is also possible for our bodies to present stress in other ways, which may at first not appear to be unrelated issues. In the final year of my PhD, I had a persistent eye twitch that simply would not go away, which I now realise was stress-related. Not an exhaustive list, but some of the physical symptoms you may encounter includes [13, 14]:

- Experiencing "brain fog", where you struggle to focus.
- Stomach aches/pains.
- Gastrointestinal issues.
- Eye twitch.
- Low libido.
- Nausea.
- Mouth ulcers.
- Eczema flares.
- Feeling dizzy.
- Panic attacks.
- Weight loss or weight gain.

Note: When experiencing physical symptoms, the first port of call should always be a medical professional. Whilst these may be caused by stress, they can also be caused by a range of other conditions.

If you recognise yourself in some of these statements, it is likely that your mental health has taken a hit. Recognising that you may need help is the first step in getting better. In Chap. 12, exactly how to get help is explored in detail.

2.4   Helping Others

Recent work by Loissel (2020) showed that 81% of PhD students have supported another PhD student with their mental health, and that 83.8% of those students were struggling with their own mental health at the time [15]. Thus, it is important to recognise the signs of mental ill-health in friends and colleagues too. I know given my own experience with mental illness, I am more compelled to help those around me, even if that is at the detriment of my own mental health.[5]

With a friend or colleague, you may notice one or several of the following [16]:

- Changes in mood.
- Withdrawal from social events.
- Lack of personal hygiene.
- Changes in behaviour.
- Seeming anxious.
- Lack of concentration.
- Changes in working hours (i.e., arriving later than typical for that person) [14].

Most important of all, is the notion that people don't pretend to be sick, typically they pretend be well.[6] In the competitive academic environment it can feel much safer to create a façade and make everyone think you are coping, even if you are not. This also means we may have friends and colleagues around us that are struggling internally, but externally to everyone else they seem absolutely fine. This can be difficult to navigate as if there are no signs of distress, there is no indication of there being a problem. This is where checking in with people directly is really useful.

We can be cautious when it comes to asking others directly about their mental health. In part, this is related to stigma, but also because it is a delicate conversation and many of us are not quite sure how best to ask how someone is really doing. The fact of the matter is you are not going to put the idea of suicide into someone's head by asking "Are you suicidal?", or "How is your mental health?" but you may give them the opportunity to open up to you.

---

[5] Putting others first may seem like the right thing to do but looking after your own mental health means that you can be well to support others. It is important to put your own oxygen mask on first.

[6] Having had conversations with people long after when I was experiencing suicidal thoughts during my PhD, I think I was incredibly good at presenting a "happy" version of myself to the world, even though I was anything but. This made it even more difficult for those around me to realise I was struggling.

Note: In some cases, a less direct approach such as "How are you feeling?", may be more appropriate, as cultural differences may also come into play where a less direct approach is preferred. This can make having conversations complex, but if in doubt: ask!

Of course, timing and location are important: it is likely better to ask questions in a private conversation not a public format. Asking someone to go for a coffee and chat with you for example may enable a 1:1 chat. It is also okay to set boundaries—when we are struggling, sometimes we do not have the capacity to help others. In this instance, encouraging someone to disclose to someone else that can help or point them in the direction of support may be the right option for you.

2.5   What Mental Health Isn't

Whilst we are discussing mental illness, I think it is also important to highlight what mental illness isn't. Given the stigma that still exists around mental health we may hear comments from those around us, including colleagues, friends, and family, based on their own biases. These can be (un)intentionally hurtful. Mental health is:

- **Not** "weakness".
- **Not** "attention seeking".
- **Not** "being lazy".
- **Not** a "poor outlook on life".
- **Not** being "stuck in a rut".
- **Not** "not trying hard enough".
- **Not** "an excuse".
- **Not** "a sin".
- **Not** "a punishment".
- **Not** "a way to avoid hard work".

And perhaps most importantly of all, mental illness is:

- **Not** your fault.

If you had a broken leg, the chances are that none of these statements would be said to you. Mental illness is exactly that—an illness—which deserves as much compassion as any other physical illness.

2.6 To Declare or Not to Declare?: That Is the Question

Choosing to declare your mental illness prior to embarking on your PhD program is a tough one. There may be benefits to acknowledging your history of mental illness ahead of time. For example, getting specific accommodations from your university to help with your studies, or simply highlighting to your PhD Supervisor that this is something you have found challenging in the past so that they know to look out for any signs you might be struggling, and provide additional support if necessary.

> Disclosing my mental illness was a relatively positive experience. My two supervisors understood things might take me a little longer and that my work would come in bursts of nothing and everything. The university itself was very helpful from helping me resit a year in undergraduate to giving me over a year of extensions for my PhD due to the Covid-19 pandemic and mental health.—PhD Student 1

Declaring can also potentially cause issues. In the United Kingdom, mental health is a protected characteristic due to the Equality Act 2010, alongside others including: age, disability, sex, sexual orientation, gender reassignment, pregnancy, marriage or civil partnership, race, religion, or belief. This makes discrimination over mental health unlawful. Yet this does not mean discrimination does not happen [17]. Further, when it comes to invisible illnesses, when declaring it, might mean you are not believed. This goes to show just how much further we have to go towards improving mental health support.

> I chose not to disclose my mental health issues for fear of being treated differently to my peers. I still to this day do not know if it was the right decision, but I think you likely know best at the time. It is important to do what feels right for you.—PhD Student 2

This makes advising declaration of mental illness difficult—it really depends on the specific circumstance you find yourself in and is ultimately your choice. Even if you cannot find support at your institution, know that there is support available to you (discussed in Chap. 12).

Now that we are up to speed with what mental health is, let's explore the "PhD Mental Health Crisis" in more detail.

References

1. World Health Organisation. Mental health: strengthening our response. https://www.who.int/news-room/fact-sheets/detail/mental-health-strengthening-our-response. Accessed 24 Jan 2022
2. Dattani S, Ritchie H, Roser M (2021) Mental health: our world in data. https://ourworldindata.org/mental-health. Accessed 24 Jan 2022
3. Mayo Clinic (2022) Mental illness. https://www.mayoclinic.org/diseases-conditions/mental-illness/symptoms-causes/syc-20374968. Accessed 24 Jan 2022
4. American Psychiatric Association (2013) Diagnostic and statistical manual of mental disorders. APA Publishing, Arlington
5. Keyes CLM (2002) The mental health continuum: from languishing to flourishing in life. J Health Soc Behav 43(2):207–222
6. Evans TM, Bira L, Gastelum JB, Weiss LT, Vanderford NL (2018) Evidence for a mental health crisis in graduate education. Nat Biotechnol 36(3):282–284
7. Schmidt CW (2007) Environmental connections: a deeper look into mental illness. Environ Health Perspect 115(8):A404–A410
8. Peay HL, Austin JC (2011) How to talk with families about genetics and psychiatric illness. Norton, New York
9. Mackie SA, Bates GW (2019) Contribution of the doctoral education environment to PhD candidates' mental health problems: a scoping review. High Educ Res Dev 38(3):565–578
10. National Alliance on Mental Illness (2022) Warning signs and symptoms. https://www.nami.org/About-Mental-Illness/Warning-Signs-and-Symptoms. Accessed 26 Jan 2022
11. Mind (2022) What are the symptoms of depression? https://www.mind.org.uk/information-support/types-of-mental-health-problems/depression/symptoms/. Accessed 26 Jan 2022
12. National Autistic Society (2022) Stimming. https://www.autism.org.uk/advice-and-guidance/topics/behaviour/stimming. Accessed 20 Jun 2022
13. Hert MDE, Correll CU, Bobes J, Cetkovich-Bakmas M, Cohen D, Asai I, Detraux J, Gautam S, Möller HJ, Ndetei DM, Newcomer JW, Uwakwe R, Leucht S (2011) Physical illness in patients with severe mental disorders. I. Prevalence, impact of medications and disparities in health care. World Psychiatr 10(1):52–77
14. Boynton P (2020) Being Well in Academia: Ways to Feel Stronger, Safer and More Connected. Routledge, Abingdon
15. Loissel E (2020) Shedding light on those who provide support. eLife 9e64739

16. Dimoff JK, Kelloway EK (2019) Signs of struggle (SOS): the development and validation of a behavioural mental health checklist for the workplace. Work Stress 33(3):295–313

17. Brouwers EPM, Mathijssen J, Van Bortel T, Knifton L, Wahlbeck K, Van Audenhove C, Kadri N, Chang C, Goud BR, Ballester D, Tófoli LF, Bello R, Jorge-Monteiro MF, Zäske H, Milaćić I, Uçok A, Bonetto C, Lasalvia A, Thornicroft G, Van Weeghel J (2016) Discrimination in the workplace, reported by people with major depressive disorder: a cross-sectional study in 35 countries. BMJ Open 6(2):e009961

3

Setting the Scene: Understanding the PhD Mental Health Crisis

Back when I started my PhD in late 2013, I did not see much discussion around PhD mental health. Thankfully, this is changing. A recent systematic review and meta-analysis of PhD student depression, anxiety, and suicidal ideation found that across the time period of 1979 to 2019, a total of 32 articles had been published talking about the so-called "PhD mental health crisis", 69% of which were published after 2015 [1, 2]. This suggests that more conversations are happening, as well as more funding being provided to support research into how to improve conditions for PhD students. I want to acknowledge that despite PhD mental health only recently coming to the fore, decades of work focusing on mental health awareness and "mad resistance", research on undergraduate mental health, as well as a broader awareness of wellbeing at work, have all paved the way to this increased (and much needed) focus on PhD mental health [3–5].

In this chapter I aim to explore these findings, and explore PhD mental health concerns, looking at the potential causes for the high incidence of mood disorders in the PhD populous. By providing you with facts and figures, my aim is to highlight how there is an unequivocal crisis happening, often silently in the background, kept out of view. In my opinion this is a systemic problem, not an individual one, thus there is an institutional responsibility to fix it.

(Trigger Warnings: suicidal ideation, suicide, self-harm, anxiety, depression, discrimination)

Z. J. Ayres, *Managing your Mental Health during your PhD*,
https://doi.org/10.1007/978-3-031-14194-2_3

3.1 Exploring the Data[1]

Looking back at the statistic that ~1 in 2 PhD students experience mental health concerns from Chap. 1, the 2014 report by UC Berkeley (one of the most cited reports to date) found that 47% of graduate students from a range of disciplines met the threshold to be considered depressed [6]. This work was expanded upon by Evans et al. (2018), finding that graduate students are more than six times as likely to experience depression and anxiety when compared to the general population (39% compared to 6% respectively for moderate to severe depression) [2]. Work by Levecque et al. (2017) [7], compared the prevalence of common mental health problems of PhD students in Belgium to a highly educated control group.[2] They found that PhD students scored more highly for twelve risk factors that increase the likelihood of mental health disorders (including feeling under constant strain, losing sleep over worry, losing confidence in self, struggling to make decisions and feeling worthless). Further, feelings of isolation, high work demands, work-life conflict, poor support, and exclusion from decision making, have all been attributed to why PhD students may experience higher incidences of mental ill-health [8].

PhD students also experience increased levels of stress and anxiety compared to the general population; a 2015 University of Arizona report found that over half of PhD students reported "more than average" stress or "tremendous" stress, during their PhD programs [9]. In the 2019 Postgraduate Research Experience Survey (PRES) spearheaded by Advance HE, only 14% of postgraduate researchers (largely PhD students) reported low levels of anxiety, compared to 41% of the general population in the UK [10]. Students also reported significantly reduced life satisfaction and happiness than the general population.

The latest biannual Nature survey (2019) [11], for PhD students in STEM subjects, also showed that PhD mental health is worsening, with 29% of respondents reporting mental health as a concern in 2017, compared to 36%

---

[1] Please note that throughout this book data that is used to discuss trends with the PhD student population is limited. It is for this reason I have chosen to use reports and research looking primarily at the PhD student experience, but also at the "researcher" experience. For these studies the majority respondents are from PhD students.

[2] Highly educated was deemed to be having successfully completed an educational program of 3–5 years outside of the university setting or having a bachelors or master's degree.

having sought help for anxiety and/or depression in 2019.[3] Although, whether this is a true rise in cases, or that reporting and discussing mental health concerns is becoming less taboo is unclear.

Mental health concerns have also worsened with the onset of the Covid-19 pandemic, with 4 in 5 researchers showing some signs of mental health distress as they navigate the pandemic [12]. If we think back to the mental health continuum model from the previous chapter, this makes sense, because with a global pandemic raging on in the background of doing a PhD, this fills up the pressure dial more, giving less space before reaching crisis point.

Sadly, suicides within the PhD population are not uncommon, though there is little formal data on prevalence.[4] I suspect the lack of data is largely to do with stigma around suicide, as well as respecting family wishes for cause of death to not be released. A study by Garcia-Williams et al. (2014) found that of a cohort of graduate students, 7.3% reported feelings of suicidal ideation, 2.3% reported plans for suicide, and 1.7% said that they had hurt themselves physically, within the last two weeks [13]. Whilst reports of suicidal ideation in the general population varies, an extensive review by Have et al. (2009) suggests that it is approximately 3% [14]. Feelings of suicidality are therefore likely higher than average for PhD students.

Another aspect that rarely gets mentioned is the drop-out rate of PhD students. This varies heavily by country, as the actual requirements for gaining a PhD also vary significantly. Discussed later on in the book, leaving a PhD program is not necessarily a bad thing—particularly when it comes to your mental health—as your wellbeing should always come first.

One of the biggest differences between PhDs in the United Kingdom (UK) compared to the United States (US), is that in the UK, PhD study has a maximum full-time study length (4 years), which can very rarely be extended beyond. In the US PhD study can be extended out much further. This difference is likely reflected in the drop-out rates observed for each country.

In the UK, little peer-reviewed data exists on program dropout rates. DiscoverPhDs.com found approximately 16.2% of PhD students "failed"[5] their PhD from 14 top universities, leaving their program before their viva [15]. So approximately 1 in 6 students never complete their PhD. In the US attrition rates range from 36 to 51% dependent on the field of study [16]. The

---

[3] Note that the 2019 survey was the first time that the survey was offered in four additional languages including Chinese, Spanish, French and Portuguese which may have impact on the results.

[4] If you are experiencing suicidal ideation and/or self-harming, there is a range of support available to you, detailed in the online resources accompanying this book.

[5] You will note I have placed "failed" in quotations. This is because I do not believe that choosing to leave a PhD is failure, it is just a different decision. We will discuss this in detail later on in the book.

fact that these drop-out rates vary institution to institution, also indicates that something else is at play—not just the incidence of mental illness in the PhD population. If there is one positive that we can take away from this though, it is that if 1 in 2 PhD students are experiencing mood disorders, many do go on and complete their PhD. Having mental illness does not define their success.

3.2   What Is the Cause?

So, what gives rise to such an extreme increase in mental health concerns among PhD students? Explanations include PhD populations being potentially predisposed to mental health concerns, where individuals with higher educational attainment[6] are more likely to introspect and self-reflect, so experience mental health concerns [17]. Intelligent individuals are also reportedly less likely to seek help [17], which is likely linked to fear of repercussions and stigma. For example, Givens and Tjia (2002) note medical students reported fear of documentation of their mental illness on their academic record, as well as lack of confidentiality [18].

Many PhD students are inadequately prepared and supported (through no fault of their own) when entering their PhD program, resulting in feelings of inadequacy and failure. In my experience, if we are not prepared by our university, and there is no forum to talk about mental health challenges, it is much harder to adapt to our new-found situation. This is in part what has inspired me to write this book—to capture the PhD experience and discuss what I wish I had known before I started.

There also may be a range of on campus support for PhD students, but that does not necessarily mean people know where to seek help. In the 2019 report by Nature, 36% of individuals reported having sought help for anxiety or depression caused by PhD study, but of these, only 26% said they got real assistance at their institution, and 9% could not find any help available [11]. This highlights that in some instances support may not be fit for purpose (for example, long waiting lists for help), or even in place to support PhD students in the first place.

---

[6] Many of these studies use IQ as a measure of intelligence, though there is evidence to suggest that IQ tests have biases, and a person can improve their IQ results over time with practice, suggesting it is not a true measure of intelligence.

3.3   Research Culture

More recently there has been a focus on another area (I would argue the most significant) that impacts mental health: **research culture**. I believe the majority of additional strain lies here, ultimately impacting PhD mental health. The way that we measure success in academia and the way that we are often forced to forgo work-life balance to get ahead, is often not conducive to maintaining good mental health. Several common themes affect the PhD student experience:

The Supervisor-PhD Student Relationship   A PhD Supervisor can make or break the PhD process. Thankfully 67% of PhD students say that they are satisfied with their PhD Supervisor relationship [11]. But when asked if they could repeat their PhD 24% of respondents stated they would choose a different PhD Supervisor. Possible explanations for this include witnessing or experiencing bullying and harassment by supervisors [19, 20]. Lack of support, not enough contact time, and not receiving positive feedback can all add strain (more on this in Chap. 9) [21]. Not receiving assistance from the very person that is supposed to guide you can have detrimental effects on wellbeing.

The Culture of Overwork   In the Nature 2019 PhD student survey, 76% of respondents reported to be working over 41+ hours per week, and approximately 5% reported working over 80 hours per week [11]. This is much higher than the EU directive (2003/88/EC) recommendations of a maximum average working week for both physical and mental health reasons [22]. In the CACTUS 2020 report "Joy and Stress Triggers: A global survey on mental health among researchers" 31% of respondents had no effective work-life balance policies in their organization and 43% did not have sufficient time for recreation/other activities [23].

Systemic Discrimination, Harassment and Microaggressions   Historically, a range of individuals, including People of Colour (POC), disabled people, women, and the LGBT+ community have been excluded by academia [24, 25]. Bullying and harassment are rife within the academy with 43% of researchers experiencing bullying and harassment, while 61% witnessed it, with women more likely (49%) to experience harassment than men (34%) [19]. This number increased when considering disabled respondents, with 62% experiencing bullying and harassment. Further, 60% of mixed race researchers and 45% of researchers identifying as homosexual reported having experienced discrimination, harassment or bullying at work [23].

The Hyper-Competitive Research Culture The research environment in academia is highly competitive, [26, 27] with 78% of researchers from the Wellcome 2020 survey suggesting that their working environment was so hyper-competitive it created "unkind and aggressive working conditions" [19]. This can be particularly problematic during the PhD process because feeling pitted against your peers, rather than being able to reach out to them for support, means that you miss out on vital help from colleagues. In a cut-throat environment, there is often a lot of fear around showing any form of "weakness", for risk of losing opportunities.

Financial Concerns Approximately 39% of PhD students are 'concerned' or 'very concerned' about debt and financial pressures, and there have been numerous studies that link debt worries with poor mental health [28]. Some PhD students may find that they are living close to a living wage, if not living on less than a living wage, due to an increase in inflation but no increase in PhD funding from funding bodies in recent years, or the precarious position of self-funding a PhD [29]. Having to pay upfront for conferences out of pocket can add further strain. International students may be particularly impacted by financial concerns with Visa stipulations affecting the possibility of taking on an extra job for financial support, or restricting the number of employment hours per week [30].

Culture of Acceptance Perhaps one of the most difficult aspects of the research culture to navigate is the culture of acceptance around struggling during a PhD. There is inherent survivor bias within academia—some that have made it to professorial positions, in my experience, tend to overlook the challenges that some individuals may face in academia because "they made it, so why can't everyone else?"

The impact of systemic issues on mental health as a PhD student is explored in detail in Part III of this book. These are often challenging situations that as a PhD student you may not be in direct control of. However, being aware of the issues you may face and the help that is available is a good place to start.

3.4   The Ups and Downs of the PhD Journey

Every PhD experience is unique. And a PhD is hard work—if it wasn't what you are studying would already be done. In a similar sense everyone's mental health journey throughout their PhD is also unique, but there are also striking similarities. To demonstrate this, I asked five individuals from a range of different disciplines to contribute their mental health journey during their PhD to Fig. 3.1. Although a simplistic way of viewing mental health during

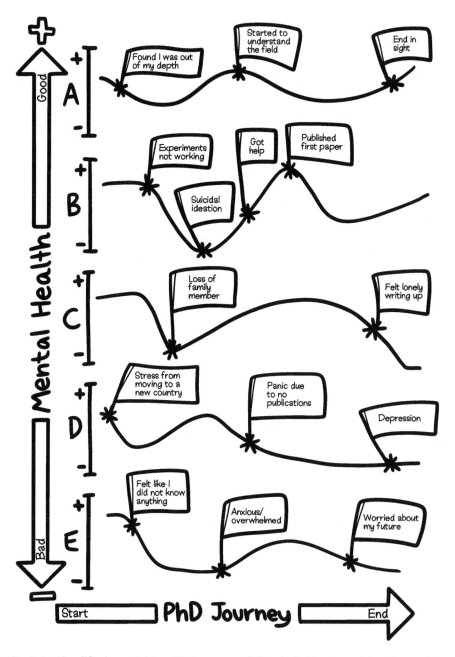

Fig. 3.1 Simplified mental health journeys of five individuals studying for a PhD, showing their mental health and how it fluctuated over their PhD study. Figure style adapted from "The PhD Experience: What they didn't tell you at induction" by Kearns et al. with permission [31]

PhD study, with some of the nuance of each journey lost, I think this is an effective way to capture the PhD experience. *Note: with mental health on the y-axis, it is fair to assume movement towards the negative means increasing likelihood of mental illness, based on the mental health continuum model discussed earlier.*

Journey A shows an individual that did not struggle notably during their PhD with their mental health. You will note there are still ups and downs as part of this person's PhD journey because there are natural highs and lows throughout life. There *will* naturally be periods where your research is more difficult. Because of these natural highs and lows, it can be difficult to pinpoint whether what you are feeling is "just part of the PhD process" or is actually part of an underlying problem. As discussed in the previous chapter, feeling low for as little as a few weeks, or experiencing suicidal ideation even once is enough to go speak to a medical professional (if available) about how you are feeling.

The other PhD mental health journeys (B-E) are all from individuals that went through periods of mental illness during their PhD, demonstrating how each experience is different. Perhaps more striking though is commonalities between PhD student experiences, going well beyond these five accounts:

Uncertainty Experiencing periods of uncertainty at the start and end of the PhD process (not knowing what to expect from the PhD process and what to expect from the world of work post-PhD respectively) is not uncommon. The fear of not knowing, can impact mental health heavily [32].

Feeling Like a Fraud Starting out on a PhD can feel like an incredible privilege (and it is). It can also make us feel like we don't deserve our position, that our PhD Supervisor has made a mistake, and that we simply are not good enough. This is impostor syndrome (or the impostor phenomenon) [33]. Feeling out of your depth at the start of your PhD is part of the learning process.[7] *Note: Other guides to starting PhD study are listed in the online resources accompanying this book.*

Pressure to Publish With academia placing value largely on publications and other metrics, this can add intense pressure on PhD students to focus on output. And to a certain extent, papers *are* currency within academia. This

---

[7] For me, it was really feeling like a fraud (struggling from the impostor phenomenon that really fuelled my struggles during my PhD. I used errors made in the lab as "proof" in my own head that I did not deserve to be doing a PhD.

can result in overworking to get ahead, ultimately leading to burnout and mental ill-health [34, 35]. In the recent CACTUS survey on researcher mental health, 65% of respondent said they were under tremendous pressure to publish papers, secure grants, and complete projects [23].

Experiencing Isolation During the PhD process, we often find ourselves working in isolation for extended periods of time, whether that is going to visit archives, during fieldwork, working from home, or writing up our thesis [36]. Social isolation can lead to increased levels of anxiety, disrupt focus, and impact sleep schedules [37–39].

Culture Shock Moving to a new town, or country can lead to experiencing feelings of isolation, as well as feeling out of your depth. Moving away from your existing support network can impact mental health. Adjusting to a new way of life can take significant time [40]. This can be particularly challenging for international students.

Feeling Overwhelmed Embarking on a PhD can feel overwhelming at throughout the process, whether it is not knowing where to start, struggling to get research outputs, or writing your thesis. Writing a thesis is effectively writing a book. This is a tough process (trust me I know!). Bringing together the last few years of research and transforming it into succinct account of what you have discovered can be a daunting task. The pressure can lead to feelings of walking away from a PhD even at such a late stage—and some people do to protect their mental health. You may experience indifference or even anger at this stage.

Managing Life Around a PhD Sometimes dedication to a PhD can be (very incorrectly) seen as at the expense of everything else, and be reinforced by academia and the inherent overwork culture. But as researchers, we are not robots. We have lives outside of our PhD programs. It can be difficult at times to juggle caring responsibilities (including looking after ourselves). Further, life events, like loss of a family member, having children, fertility problems, health problems, and moving house, can all add additional strain [41]. This can impact mental health, particularly when there is the background pressure of making sure that enough research is generated within a certain time period to get a PhD.

Studying a Topic That You Care Deeply About In some cases, what motivated you to go into a particular research area may be linked to your own personal experiences. For example, understanding eating disorders or documenting the experiences of survivors of violence. Thus, researching topics we care passionately about can impact us heavily and sometimes unexpectedly [42]. If you find there is little professional support available at your institution, this can make studying these topics difficult.

In my journey, it was the breaking of a piece of very expensive equipment that really triggered a cascade downward of my mental health. Whilst the experimental mishap I had was not preventable, I used it to evidence to myself that I was a *real* impostor, and not cut out for research.

3.5   There Is Hope

Now, despite all the statistics presented in this chapter, it doesn't necessarily mean all PhD students do not enjoy the work that they do. In the 2019 Advance HE Postgraduate Research Experience Survey over 80% of students were positive about their research experience [10]. Further, in the Nature 2019 survey 38% of students said that they were very satisfied with their decision to embark on a PhD, and 75% said they were at least somewhat satisfied [11]. It can be inferred that many students who have mental illness(es) still enjoy their research.

It is also important to realise that just because these statistics exist, doesn't mean struggling with your mental health is going to happen to *you* [43]. Your situation, the support you have available, and your ability to be resilient and survive, even when there is little scope to do so, is unique. It also certainly does not mean that those of us that have mental illness are being set up to fail. Instead, it means that we may need to be aware of the support that is available to us to help us navigate the process.

Throughout the remainder of the book, I will challenge you and your mindset in places, to help bolster your resilience and prepare you for your PhD journey. Further, what I cannot do is change all the systemic issues throughout academia that exist. I can, however, highlight them, like a lighthouse shining bright in a storm, so you know what dangers lie ahead and what to avoid. In some cases, avoidance will not be possible. In these instances, I will provide you with tips and tricks to best navigate the challenges ahead.

References

1. Satinsky EN, Kimura T, Kiang MV, Abebe R, Cunningham S, Lee H, Lin X, Liu CH, Rudan I, Sen S, Tomlinson M, Yaver M, Tsai AC (2021) Systematic review and meta-analysis of depression, anxiety, and suicidal ideation among Ph.D. students. Sci Rep 11(1):14370
2. Evans TM, Bira L, Gastelum JB, Weiss LT, Vanderford NL (2018) Evidence for a mental health crisis in graduate education. Nat Biotechnol 36(3):282–284
3. Bertolote J (2008) The roots of the concept of mental health. World Psychiatry 7(2):113–116
4. Crook S (2020) Historicising the "crisis" in undergraduate mental health: British universities and student mental illness, 1944–1968. J Hist Med Allied Sci 75(2):193–220
5. Andersen J, Altwies E, Bossewitch J, Brown C, Cole K, Davidow S, DuBrul SA, Friedland-Kays E, Fontaine G, Hall W, Hansen C, Lewis B, Mitchell-Brody M, McNamara J, Nikkel G, Sadler P, Stark D, Utah A, Vidal A, Weber CL (2017) Mad resistance/mad alternatives: democratizing mental health care. In: Community mental health. Routledge, Abingdon
6. The Graduate Assembly (2014) Graduate student happiness & well-being report. University of California, Berkeley, CA
7. Levecque K, Anseel F, De Beuckelaer A, Van der Heyden J, Gisle L (2017) Work organization and mental health problems in PhD students. Res Policy 46(4):868–879
8. Guthrie S, Lichten C, Belle J, Ball S, Knack A, Hofman J (2017) Understanding mental health in the research environment. RAND Europe, Cambridge, UK
9. Smith E, Brooks Z (2015) Graduate student mental health. University of Arizona Tucson, AZ
10. Williams S (2019) Postgraduate research experience survey 2019. Advance HE, York
11. Woolston C (2019) PhDs: the tortuous truth. Nature 575(7782):403–407
12. Byrom N (2020) The challenges of lockdown for early-career researchers. eLife:9e59634
13. Garcia-Williams AG, Moffitt L, Kaslow NJ (2014) Mental health and suicidal behavior among graduate students. Acad Psychiatry 38:554–560
14. ten Have M, De Graaf R, Van Dorsselaer S, Verdurmen J, Van't Land H, Vollebergh W, Beekman A (2009) Incidence and course of suicidal ideation and suicide attempts in the general population. Can J Psychiatry 54(12):824–833
15. DiscoverPhDs (2017) PhD failure rate – a study of 26,076 PhD candidates. https://www.discoverphds.com/advice/doing/phd-failure-rate.   Accessed 3 Mar 2022
16. Young SN, Vanwye WR, Schafer MA, Robertson TA, Poore AV (2019) Factors affecting PhD student success. Int J Exerc Sci 12(1):34–45

17. Karpinski RI, Kolb AMK, Tetreault NA, Borowski TB (2018) High intelligence: a risk factor for psychological and physiological overexcitabilities. Intelligence: 668–623

18. Givens JL, Tjia J (2002) Depressed medical students' use of mental health services and barriers to use. Acad Med 77(9):918–921

19. Moran H, Karlin L, Lauchlan E, Rappaport SJ, Bleasdale B, Wild L, Dorr J (2020) Understanding research culture: what researchers think about the culture they work in. Wellcome Trust, London, UK

20. Moss SE, Mahmoudi M (2021) STEM the bullying: an empirical investigation of abusive supervision in academic science. EClinicalMedicine 40:101121

21. Devos C, Boudrenghien G, Van der Linden N, Azzi A, Frenay M, Galand B, Klein O (2017) Doctoral students' experiences leading to completion or attrition: a matter of sense, progress and distress. Eur J Psychol Educ 32(1):61–77

22. Limas JC, Corcoran LC, Baker AN, Cartaya AE, Ayres ZJ (2022) The impact of research culture on mental health & diversity in STEM. Chemistry s(9):e202102957

23. Cerejo C, Awati M, Hayward A (2020) Joy and stress triggers: a global survey on mental health among researchers. CACTUS Foundation, Solapur

24. Berhe AA, Barnes RT, Hastings MG, Mattheis A, Schneider B, Williams BM, Marín-Spiotta E (2022) Scientists from historically excluded groups face a hostile obstacle course. Nat Geosci 15(1):2–4

25. Bhopal K (2015) The experiences of black and minority ethnic academics: a comparative study of the unequal academy. Routledge, Abingdon

26. Woolston C (2018) Feeling overwhelmed by academia? You are not alone. Nature 557(7706):129–131

27. Moore S, Neylon C, Eve MP, Paul O'Donnell D, Pattinson D (2017) "Excellence R Us": university research and the fetishisation of excellence. Palgrave Commun 3:16105

28. Russo G (2013) Education: financial burden. Nature 501(7468):579–581

29. Khoo S (2021) How Canada short-changes its graduate students and postdocs. https://www.universityaffairs.ca/opinion/in-my-opinion/how-canada-short-changes-its-graduate-students-and-postdocs/. Accessed 4 Mar 2022

30. UK Council for International Student Affairs (2022) Student work. https://www.ukcisa.org.uk/Information%2D%2DAdvice/Working/Student-work. Accessed 2 Jun 2022

31. Kearns H, Gardiner M, Marchall K, Banytis F (2006) The PhD experience: what they didn't tell you at induction. ThinkWell, Glenelg North

32. Jackman PC, Jacobs L, Hawkins RM, Sisson K (2021) Mental health and psychological wellbeing in the early stages of doctoral study: a systematic review. Eur J High Educ. 12(3):293–313

33. Clance PR, Imes SA (1978) The imposter phenomenon in high achieving women: dynamics and therapeutic intervention. Psychother Theory Res Pract 15(3):241–247

34. De Rond M, Miller AN (2005) Publish or perish: bane or boon of academic life? J Manage Inq 14(4):321–329
35. Miller AN, Taylor SG, Bedeian AG (2011) Publish or perish: academic life as management faculty live it. Career Development International. Emerald, Bingley, UK
36. Hazell CM, Chapman L, Valeix SF, Roberts P, Niven JE, Berry C (2020) Understanding the mental health of doctoral researchers: a mixed methods systematic review with meta-analysis and meta-synthesis. Syst Rev 9(1):197
37. Lim MH, Rodebaugh TL, Zyphur MJ, Gleeson JFM (2016) Loneliness over time: the crucial role of social anxiety. J Abnorm Psychol 125(5):620–630
38. Yu B, Steptoe A, Niu K, Ku P, Chen L (2018) Prospective associations of social isolation and loneliness with poor sleep quality in older adults. Qual Life Res 27(3):683–691
39. Casey C, Harvey O, Taylor J, Knight F, Trenoweth S (2022) Exploring the well-being and resilience of postgraduate researchers. J Further High Educ 46(6):850–867
40. Zapf MK (1991) Cross-cultural transitions and wellness: dealing with culture shock. Int J Adv Couns 14(2):105–119
41. Sokratous S, Merkouris A, Middleton N, Karanikola M (2013) The association between stressful life events and depressive symptoms among Cypriot university students: a cross-sectional descriptive correlational study. BMC Public Health 13(1):1121
42. Dickson-Swift V, James EL, Kippen S, Liamputtong P (2007) Doing sensitive research: what challenges do qualitative researchers face? Qual Res 7(3):327–353
43. Boynton P (2020) Being Well in Academia: Ways to Feel Stronger, Safer and More Connected. Routledge, Abingdon

Part II

Mindset Matters

4

Self-Care: Without You There Is No PhD

I strongly considered whether or not I wanted to include this chapter at all. So often in my experience, wellbeing advice is simply built around self-care and nothing more for PhD students, focusing solely on what individuals "can do better", how to maintain a "positive mindset", or manage stress through a myriad of potential issues. This was in itself a major source of frustration during my own PhD as there is so much more to the PhD experience and what might impact mental health than if we "eat right" or not. However, I have concluded over time that self-care has huge value as a tool to make the PhD experience more manageable, and absolutely has a place in this book. I see investment in self-care as the shoring up of our foundations so that we increase our chance of success.

When I first heard the phrase "self-care", I remember thinking I wanted absolutely nothing to do with it. I was there to do a PhD, not sing "Kumbaya" in a group or meditate.[1] I didn't have time for that—there was research to be done, and I was a scientist with 'no tolerance for rubbish'. If this is you right now, I want to spend some time convincing you that investing in yourself is the biggest, most important thing you can do for yourself *and* your PhD research. Simply put—I was wrong. If you have already come to this realisation and you are already on your self-care journey, I hope you can find

---

(Trigger warnings: Eating Disorders, Addiction)

---

[1] Meditation really doesn't work for me (I find my brain is "too loud" for me to relax into it), but this doesn't mean it is not a valuable and important tool for some to improve wellbeing. Different people find comfort in different self-care practises.

yourself mirrored in this chapter and use it to feel good about putting yourself first.

Self-care, as defined by the World Health Organisation is "the ability of individuals, families and communities to promote health, prevent disease, maintain health, and to cope with illness and disability with or without the support of a healthcare provider" [1]. In other words, by engaging in self-care we are committing to look after ourselves both mentally and physically. This can reduce stress; help improve our resilience; and help us manage pre-existing mental illness(es). Self-care helps us improve our *capacity to cope* with whatever comes our way.

So, why should we care about self-care as PhD researchers? For me, it is simple. In the pursuit of academic excellence, we must look after our own wellbeing. To neglect ourselves is to not bring our A-game, meaning we have no energy left to give to the research that we love. To be the best researchers we can be we must put ourselves first, as without us, there would be no research. In this sense looking after our mental health aligns well with the main aims and objectives of the academy as it enables us to: publish high impact papers, obtain intellectual property, get research featured (positively) in the news etc. However, the link between wellbeing and output is not always respected. Often the 'culture of overwork' commonly associated with academia means that the preference from our institutions is that we work like machines, powering on through irrespective of how we feel, never stopping to question if we are physically or mentally well enough to be doing our research [2]. This must change, and it is—slowly.

The first step in understanding self-care as a PhD student is that we are not robots. We cannot simply ignore our health. Self-care is essential to long-term, sustainable progress during our PhD. Pushing too hard may mean reaching burnout, which as PhD researchers can make us unwell, having a knock-on impact on our PhD studies [3].

According to the International Classification of Diseases, "burnout" is an "occupational phenomenon" and can be defined as: "A syndrome conceptualised as resulting from chronic workplace stress that has not been successfully managed, characterised by three factors:

- feelings of energy depletion or exhaustion;
- increased mental distance from one's job, or feelings of negativism or cynicism related to one's job; and
- reduced professional efficacy" [4].

If possible, clearly, this is something that is best avoided. Self-care is one of the ways to do this.

One of the first things to know about self-care is that it is a huge learning journey. It also may evolve over time—one thing that works for you at one time point in your life might not work for you in another. For example, many people use physical exercise to release endorphins and relieve stress, [5] but what would happen if you were to break your leg suddenly? Your self-care would have to adapt accordingly.[2] It is therefore important to recognise that self-care needs to be adaptable, and is different person to person, depending on needs and circumstance. It is therefore sensible to consider what your self-care routine looks like and diversify if needed.

Note, there is a darker side of self-care. When workloads are higher than they should be, or pressures too much, there is often a push towards individualism when it comes to mental health: that we must be more resilient, lean more heavily on self-care, and power on through. This is not okay. There is only so much anyone should have to deal with at any given time. Thus, self-care is a valuable tool, but every tool has it's limit.

4.1   Setting the Foundations

In all likelihood, you have probably heard advice on eating well, doing physical exercise, and getting enough sleep a hundred times before. It is certainly not my intention to only talk about what *you* can do to maintain good mental health throughout this book. In my opinion, this information is routinely reiterated to us by university wellbeing programs, in part because it is a relatively simple way to provide general wellbeing advice (more on this in the next chapter) but also put the fault on us if we do not stay well. And whilst I fundamentally disagree with this approach (I believe systemic issues in the academy must be addressed) it is essential that we realise that mastering these "foundations of wellbeing" can really help with managing our mental health. For this reason, I will spend some time discussing why they are important and how you might make these work for you as a busy PhD student.

I want to recognise that it is easy for me to dish out this advice, but there may be a range of factors *outside your control*, that affect your self-care. For this section focus is placed on what you *can* control. You may not be able to do everything. That is more than okay. If self-care itself ultimately is causing you more distress, it may be time to step away from it.

---

[2] This did in fact happen to me, which is part of the reason I am writing this book right now.

4.2   Establishing a Good Sleep Schedule

Several studies have shown that doctoral students have a reduced night's sleep on average, compared to the recommended 7–9 hours' sleep, [6] averaging around 6.4 hours sleep [7]. At first glance, looking at these numbers you may think, "the difference between 7 and 6.4 hours of sleep is negligible", but even slightly less sleep than we need can impact our behaviour and our mental health. Lack of sleep (struggling with insomnia) has also been linked with increased likelihood of anxiety, stress, and depression [8].

Further, lack of sleep may directly impact your PhD work. You may feel more fatigued during your work day, be irritable, lose interest in activities that usually bring you joy, and lack of concentration may lead to reduced work quality. Problem-solving and decision making has also been found to be affected, even after just one night of lost sleep [9]. Thus it is important to consider whether an "all-nighter" is truly worth it for your overall productivity. Long-term, investment in sleep is key.

> **Task**
>
> Ask yourself: *Are you actually getting enough sleep?* If you do not know the answer to this question, I task you with monitoring your sleep for a week. You can use fancy gadgets such as sleep monitoring watches, but in reality, you can make an approximation through writing down the time you switch off your bedroom light to sleep, noting down if you wake up in the night, and what time you wake up. If by the end of the week you find that you are not getting the required 7–9 hours of sleep, it may be time to rethink your sleep schedule. This is where establishing good sleep hygiene comes in.

Sleep hygiene is a series of **active** steps that you can take to improve the quality and quantity of your sleep [10]. It requires effort to implement some of these changes to start with, but with time they are likely to become part of your everyday routine. Some examples of changes you could make include:

Regulating Caffeine Intake Caffeine is a stimulant and can remain in the body for quite some time (a single dose of caffeine has a half-life of 3–7 hours) [11]. It may not be realistic (or desirable) to cut out caffeine entirely, but consider decaffeinated options in the afternoon.

Reducing Screen Time Before Bed[3] Light from our devices, such as phones, TVs, and laptops can make it more difficult to sleep, as it can affect our circadian rhythm and impact melatonin production that helps us sleep [12]. Consider not using artificially lit devices an hour before you intend to sleep. One effective way of avoiding using your phone is charging it at a plug socket across the other side of your room.

Getting Exposure to Natural Light Natural light helps calibrate our circadian rhythm, helping our body determine the time of day it is and when to sleep [13]. If natural light is not possible (for example due to the latitude of where you live), light exposure/light therapy during the day may help.

Try to Avoid Working from Your Bed Not always possible[4] (you may live in a studio apartment for example or suffer from chronic illness which means working from bed is easier for you), keeping your bed as a dedicated sleeping space, and not using it to work can help you mentally switch off at night by associating the space with sleeping.

Aim to Go to Bed at the Same Time Each Night Establishing a routine and set time that you go to bed can help prepare your body for a good night's sleep. This is not always possible due to deadlines, or simply wanting to have a night out with friends but aiming to be consistent the majority of the week will help.

Establish a Relax Routine Commit to doing relaxing activities before bed. This could be having a cup of herbal tea, reading a book, crafting, taking a bath, meditating, or anything else that helps you unwind that you have access to [14].

Write Down Your Worries Sometimes we can struggle to turn our thoughts and anxieties off when trying to sleep. A tip is to have a notebook by your bed that you can write these concerns into to help put them aside until the morning.

---

[3] I am particularly bad for not doing this, as those of you that follow me on Twitter will know. I wanted to comment on this to show that whilst I am giving this advice, implementing it is hard. I am certainly not perfect even though I know what *would* be best for me.

[4] Or like me, some days you might be struggling with your mental health and try as you might you find it difficult if not impossible to get out of bed. On these days I now tend to work from my bed, snuggled in my duvet (it makes me feel much better) and is a worthwhile trade-off for me when it comes to sleep hygiene versus managing my depression for the day.

If you try these sleep hygiene activities and you are still struggling with sleep, I advise you go speak to a medical professional if you have access. They can help you figure out why your sleep is being impacted and help you work towards a healthier sleep cycle. Know that you will not always get your sleep "right", but you can reset and start working towards better sleep hygiene at any time.

4.3   Eat Nutritious Food

You are all adults, so I am not going to spend long on telling you the importance of eating nutritious food. You will likely have heard it before. I'm also not going to presume to tell you what eating "well" looks like for you. I am not a nutritionist so am not qualified to give you specific advice on what you should or shouldn't be eating.

Eating well can however make a difference during your PhD. Eating regularly can enable you to maintain focus, as can drinking adequate amounts of water [15, 16]. If you tend to forget to drink during the day[5] setting a reminder on your phone to drink or getting a drinking bottle with demarcated lines on it may help. Keeping snacks on hand to help fuel you when you have an energy low may be also useful. *Tip: If you routinely forget to eat or skip meals, making eating a social event, for example sharing cooking meals with friends or flat mates across the week, can keep you accountable.*

Financial difficulties can also make "eating well" tough, such as being able to afford fresh ingredients and expensive proteins like meat and fish. Bulk buying ingredients like pasta and rice and getting proteins through a largely vegetarian diet for a while can help cost save (though having the money to bulk buy can be a privilege in itself). *Tip: Please see additional resources link at the back of the book for more support.*

When we are under stress, eating can become a way for us to try to maintain control. This can manifest as eating disorders such as anorexia nervosa, bulimia nervosa or binge eating disorder. Lipson et al. (2017) studied both undergraduate and graduate populations, finding 11% of students had an elevated eating disorder risk, and 40.2% of students had engaged in binge-eating behaviours in the last month [17]. It was also found that individuals that identified as LGBTQ+, were more likely to have an eating disorder.

Eating disorders are challenging to recover from and can be deadly if left unchecked. If you are struggling at the moment, first: well done for

---

[5] As a laboratory scientist I can forget to drink for several hours straight which I know is not good for me, and I know this, yet I still forget!

acknowledging there might be a problem (this is the first step to recovery). Second, know there is help available for you, including speaking to a medical professional. You are not alone.

There has also been some studies linking low Vitamin D (from sunlight) to mental illnesses, including depression [18]. Whilst there are some dietary sources of Vitamin D, most Vitamin D is made from getting sunlight on our skin when outdoors. As PhD students, taking less vacation and staying inside to study, the lifestyle often means working indoors in offices and/or labs for extended periods. Thus, taking the time to ensure that you are getting the right nutrition is important, and it may be a good idea to consider taking vitamin supplements (in the UK governmental advice is to take a Vitamin D supplement in Autumn and Winter) [19]. Of course, this advice may be different, depending on your country of study.

4.4   Physical Exercise

There is often inherent ableism that exists within any wellbeing advice that suggests to "just get out end exercise more". From experience, being told to do physical exercise when you can't, can itself affect mental health. You may not be able to do physical exercise for a variety of reasons, but please do not worry, because if you cannot it doesn't mean that you cannot get a "complete" self-care routine. Further, for those of you working part-time on a PhD, to those of you with caring responsibilities, finding the time to exercise can be a challenge. We should not be made to feel shamed for not being able to find the time.

For those that can, physical exercise has been shown to improve physical health and reduce risk of major illnesses such as stroke, heart disease, type II diabetes and cancer. It also has huge benefits for our mental health. Research has shown that exercise can improve cognitive function and academic performance [20].

Fitting physical exercise in around a busy PhD schedule is possible by:

Establishing a Routine You are more likely to stick to your exercise plan if you establish a routine and stick with it. Even 10 minutes a day is better than no exercise, and research has found that high intensity, short burst exercise is just as effective as medium intensity exercise, over a longer time period (good to know if you are time strapped!) [21]. *Tip: It can take a few weeks to really get into a routine so stick at it.*

Finding a Sport You Enjoy If like me, you were forced to do a whole host of sports you didn't enjoy at school, know that there is a sport out there for you. The university setting provides a unique opportunity to try different sports and activities through university clubs. This is also a great way to meet new friends.

Realising It Does Not Have to Be Expensive There is a tendency to think that we need fancy gym memberships in order to exercise, when in reality we can do cheaper alternatives of exercises using water bottles for weights and YouTube videos for fitness plan ideas if needed.

4.5   Managing Finances

Not often mentioned in self-care, managing finances can make a huge difference to wellbeing, and financial hardship is not uncommon for PhD students, with a recent 2020 SERU survey of US graduate students revealing that 19% of graduate students experienced food insecurity [22]. Further, approximately 1 in 5 PhD students have an additional job alongside their PhD, with 53% of them doing them to make ends meet [23].

With the tips to help manage financial hardship that follow, I want to highlight that whilst these are a place to start, I do not wish to suggest that financial struggles are easy and straightforward to manage, and that if you just follow my advice, you will be fine. I acknowledge financial strains can be huge barriers. Juggling several part-time jobs on top of PhD research is a huge feat and is likely going to impact other aspects of self-care (for example simply not having the time or energy for some activities). Further, managing your finances (however well) is not going to make up for the chronic underfunding of PhD studentships and in some cases lack of a living wage, and it certainly cannot make more money when there is none. If you are struggling with money, it is also highly likely that you will be surrounded by colleagues that have never had to worry about their finances. This is one of the many reasons why comparing your PhD journey to others is not helpful. Know that completing your PhD in spite of having financial difficulties is a huge achievement. *Note: If you feel you are disadvantaged by your financial situation, speaking to your PhD Supervisor or course coordinator is a great place to start.*

Planning your finances can be hugely helpful. This might include creating an Excel spreadsheet of your spending for a month. By doing this you may be able to identify areas where you are spending more than you are budgeting for and can adjust accordingly. If you find that even after planning, you are struggling financially, there are options available to you:

Hardship Funds Most universities have a student hardship fund (or similar) available for students to apply for if they are in financial difficulty. More recently, professional bodies (such as the Royal Society of Chemistry and their Chemists' Community Fund) are also providing financial support.

Studying Part-Time PhD study does not have to be full-time and can be split over a longer period of time. This enables study around another job to be able to have financial security. This is also a popular option for PhD students with chronic illness. The possibility of doing part-time work is often dependent on grant stipulations, and may not be possible on some Visas.

Getting a Part-Time Job It may be possible to get a part-time job (or several) around your PhD. Managing this can be incredibly tough. Possible ways to complement your PhD, is considering jobs such as tutoring, proof-reading, or writing for relevant magazines. There may be extra teaching you can do at your university to make extra cash. *Note: This may not be possible due to Visa stipulations in some situations.*

Food Banks If you find you are struggling to make ends meet and this is impacting your ability to afford food, country-dependent there are often local food banks and soup kitchens that can give you a free meal. Faith-based organisations may be of assistance. It is important to inform your graduate school if you are struggling to the extent of needing food banks for survival, as there may be more support (or at least understanding of your situation) available.

4.6   Examples of Self-Care

The range of self-care options are huge, and I cannot summarise them all here, but for me they divide into clear categories, shown in Table 4.1.

Task

Think about your current self-care routine (or lack of). What could you build into your daily life? If you do not already, it may be beneficial to add your self-care activities to your calendar, log them in a diary, or use an app to log them.

Examples of different types of self-care [24]

f-care	Examples
...ar	• Exercising
	• Taking medication
	• Sleep
	• Stretching
	• Rest
	• Meal preparation
	• Hygiene
Emotional	• Practicing mindfulness
	• Therapy
Spiritual	• Meditation
	• Worship
	• Reducing screen time
Creativity	• Hobbies
	• Reading
	• Journaling
Financial	• Paying bills
	• Budgeting
	• Meal Planning
Social	• Meeting friends
	• Communication
	• Spending time with family
	• Establishing boundaries
	• Spending time alone

4.7 Putting Self-Care in Context of a PhD

Now we have explored what self-care is, I want to explore how to establish a self-care routine around your PhD work. As a PhD student you will be busy and prioritising your wellbeing may inadvertently be affected. It can seem counterproductive to take time out of doing your PhD work to look after your wellbeing, but only by doing so can you ensure that you are prepared and ready for what is a long distance run not a short sprint. So how might you do this?

Acknowledge That There Will Always Be more Work to Be Done The open-ended nature of PhD study can make us feel like we need to always be working to succeed, particularly in the first few years of a PhD where we feel out of our depth because we know little about our field of study. It is important to realise there is always more work that *could* be done, it doesn't mean it *should* be done straight away. Building knowledge takes time.

Prioritise Self-Care When Things Get Tough As tempting as it can be when we have a looming deadline to cease all self-care activities to deliver on what is required of us, we need to resist doing this. Taking half an hour out to look after yourself is likely not going to impede you. In fact, taking a moment to for you can actually help you be more efficient.

Schedule in Time for Self-Care In your work diary, schedule in routine times that you might engage in some self-care activities. Maybe this would be ensuring you always take a lunch break and go for a walk three times a week during that lunch break. *Tip: If you do not have full autonomy over your schedule (for example your PhD Supervisor is prone to scheduling last minute meetings) consider taking your self-care time in lieu and move it to a different time in the day.*

Understand That It Does Not Have to Be Time or Money Intensive When we think of self-care we can often think of time or money intensive activities like going for a half an hour walk or booking on to a spa day. You can take a shorter period of time to reset your thoughts through mindfulness practices, for example, taking a minute to close your eyes and relax, which will still help support your wellbeing. *Tip: Consider building self-care into meetings. Could meetings be 50 minutes long not 1 hour in order for attendees to have a break between meetings (for any meetings you have direct control over)?*

Think About Time-Saving Options If time is tight, there are self-care tasks you can do to help yourself. For example, meal prepping for the week can be both time and cost saving. Could you combine your exercise for the day in with your commute? If you are driving to work, could you park in a car park slightly further away to get more of a walk in? Could you limit working out of hours (If you feel you have to) to only some evenings of the week so you can ensure you also practice self-care?

Realise What Works for You as Self-Care Might Change During Your PhD Anecdotally, one of the issues I often see PhD students struggle with is reading for pleasure. Before starting a PhD, this might have been useful self-care, but given the intensity of a PhD program and the sheer volume of reading required, often there is no energy or motivation left to do this. This means that other forms of self-care might need to be explored.[6]

---

[6] Personally, it has taken me about 4 years post-PhD to pick up a novel and actually read it. It was Leviathan Wakes by James S. A. Corey, if you are interested! For a long while I was reading non-fiction to "better myself" rather than reading for actual enjoyment.

You Will Likely Get It Wrong PhD's can be unpredictable, with periods of high intensity and low intensity. This means that your self-care may have to adapt to the current situation you find yourself in. It is a learning process so you will not get everything "right" all the time. *Tip: Remember you can hit the "reset button" on self-care at any time. You don't have to wait for next week to start again.*

If you are really struggling to even comprehend having the energy to engage with self-care, this may be indicative of you struggling with your mental health. This is reason enough to consider speaking to a medical professional.

4.8   Acknowledging There May Be a Problem: Addiction

As discussed earlier in this chapter, self-care helps us improve our capacity to cope with whatever comes our way and is particularly useful throughout the PhD process. There are, however, other ways we might improve our capacity to cope that can ultimately be dangerous for our health. This includes taking drugs or drinking alcohol to excess. Although often associated with undergraduate students, Cranford et al. (2009), found that approximately 34% of graduate students had engaged in binge drinking behaviours in the last 2 weeks [25].

At first, you may think that these substances may help you release stress, but long-term heavy use can have health consequences. They may also lead you to end up in situations where you are in danger or extremely vulnerable and can result in monetary trouble due to financing these habits.

> **Task**
>
> Think about your drinking habits—are you drinking alcohol more than you used to or using it (excessively) as a way to relax? With alcohol specifically it is also easy to let the amount we drink creep up over time, and not necessarily register that we are drinking more than we used to. The recommended maximum amount of alcohol consumption varies country to country and should be used as a healthy guideline.

One of the biggest forms of self-care is setting boundaries for ourselves. We have a finite amount of energy and exceeding beyond this can lead to increased strain, add stress, and result in us neglecting our self-care. Setting boundaries can be one of the most difficult things we can do but is perhaps the most important. This is reflected in the number of fantastic books on setting boundaries out there, that are well worth checking out if you struggle to put yourself first [27, 28]. Setting boundaries is important in the working environment just as much as in our personal relationships, as poor boundaries can lead to feelings of resentment, anger (towards others as well as internalised), and ultimately burnout.

Before we explore setting boundaries, it is therefore important to understand that:

You Can Be Your Own Saboteur Enthusiasm can be our best friend, but it can also lead to overcommitment. By not planning your time you may find yourself overburdened.

It Might Not Be "Good for Your Career" We can justify taking on more and more extracurricular activities because it will help advance our career. However, if you are overstretched, it may mean that you let the ball drop, and do not deliver quality work. Ultimately that "one more thing" you get involved in is unlikely to benefit you as much as you think it might, so concentrating on a few manageable tasks may be more useful.

People May Not Have Your Best Interests at Heart When people ask you to do additional labour that pushes you to the brink in order to deliver, they often have a vested interest in doing so and may not have even considered your wellbeing. This may not be done with malice, but they may need a reminder. *Tip: Remember that one person's lack of organisation is not your urgency.*

Choosing to Set a Boundary Might Not Be Black or White In some situations, setting a boundary may help you slightly (for example protect your time), but it may also help someone else out. For example, helping a friend with an outreach program. In these situations, we may choose to bend these boundaries to support those around us, or choose to be honest with our friend to ensure they understand why helping would stretch us too thin.

Boundary Setting Is Not Lack of Kindness Sometimes we must prioritise ourselves. Individuals looking to make you feel guilty for setting boundaries may not be as supportive as you originally thought. Boundary setting is often the biggest act of kindness we can show *ourselves*.

Setting Boundaries to Protect Your Health Are Non-negotiable There is a culture of presenteeism in academia, which in reality leads to people feeling like they cannot take time off when sick. However, when you are ill, you are likely to make your illness last longer if not getting sufficient rest. Saying you are ill and that you will not be working is a more than acceptable and essential boundary.

So practically, during your PhD program how do you set boundaries during your PhD?

To reiterate the name of this chapter "without you there is no PhD". To have time to look after your mental health you must set boundaries. Yet, given the hyper-competitive nature of academia and the culture of overwork, it can feel difficult to take a step back and set boundaries for fear of missing out. Knowing where your boundary limits are is trial and error, and something we learn over time.

Know It Is Okay to Not Reply Immediately We can feel compelled to respond to requests immediately (particularly to our PhD Supervisors due to the power dynamic that exists—more on this in Chap. 9). In fact, it has been found that as receivers of emails we often overestimate how quickly the sender expect us to respond to non-urgent emails and that this stress can impact wellbeing [29]. In short: we often don't actually need to respond as quickly as we think we do. If you receive correspondence outside of work hours you are entitled to delay responding to the following day. *Tip: do not be afraid to use the phrase "let me check my schedule and get back to you" if you are placed on the spot during a conversation.*

Consider Deleting Your Work Emails Off Your Phone Having clear physical boundaries between your home life and work life, like not having your university emails on your personal phone can help create separation. *Tip: Remember that most of the time the work will wait until tomorrow.*

Do Not Feel You Have to Justify When setting boundaries we can often feel the need to give a reason. You do not have to. For example, wanting to have work-life balance and not work your evenings because you have children and want to spend time with them is just as valid as not having children and wanting to relax in your evenings. You do not have to justify your personal life.

Set Your Own Deadlines If someone is asking you to produce work quickly but you know that the work is going to take longer, be honest, and provide feedback. Give them a realistic turnaround time based on your schedule.

Say "No" More Say "no" to opportunities straight away if you want to but allow yourself some thinking time before you say yes to something. By waiting a short while you will not miss the opportunity, but you may realise you do not have the capacity to take another project on.

Think About Future You When saying "yes" to new opportunities we can do so with enthusiasm, but we must consider our time and energy as resources. Whilst you have the energy now, do you have the energy to commit to something three months in the future?

Be Kind to Yourself Setting boundaries takes a lot of practice, and even if you have been effectively setting boundaries for a while it is still more than likely that you will get your boundary setting wrong from time to time.

A final note on setting boundaries and self-care is that circumstance can result in us not having the flexibility or privilege to say "no" to working weekends (or outside of shift patterns). For example, self-funding a PhD may mean that you are committed to finishing your PhD as quickly as possible. Further, if you need additional teaching work or to bring in research grants to make

---

Saying "no" can be hard, so here are some examples of what you could say to help you set boundaries and prioritise opportunities:

- Thank you for the opportunity. Unfortunately, I am at capacity right now and cannot commit to taking on another project. *(Honest and to the point)*.
- Please can you confirm if this is a paid opportunity? *(Seeing if an offer is a paid opportunity can help you prioritise)*.
- I could take this work on but given that I am running at capacity right now, I suspect the work I would deliver would not be to the standard that you and this project deserves. *(Being honest can help reiterate your point, and not many people are then going to force you to take on a project you have said you likely will under-deliver on)*.
- Please ask me again in a week. My schedule should hopefully have cleared up by then.
- I would not be able to do this for another [insert time period]. *(Both setting clear, realistic time boundaries)*.

---

ends meet and pay bills, slowing down may seem impossible. In these situations, prioritising what is best for you (for example focusing on paid work) is even more essential. It is important to remember that prioritising yourself is not selfish, it is self-preservation.

4.10 What to Do If You Reach Burnout

As discussed at the start of this chapter burnout is best avoided, but unfortunately, we may not always manage this. If you have hit burnout, this is not a fault with you. Learning to balance workload, set boundaries, and saying "no" takes time and experience. Some of the signs of burnout include [30, 31]:

- Disconnect from work/loss of motivation
- Physical and/or emotional exhaustion
- Difficulty concentrating
- Drop in creativity
- Withdrawal from socialising
- Feelings of hopelessness
- Feeling overwhelmed by workload
- Work quality decline
- Feelings of anxiety/depression

Recognising these in ourselves is often easier said than done. We can think that we are simply not good enough and that is why we are struggling, when in reality no person could be functioning well with the level of stress and workload we are under.

One of the biggest barriers to realising we are experiencing burnout is thinking that a PhD is "meant to be hard", so what you are experiencing is normal. However, there is a difference between your PhD being challenging, and your PhD damaging your physical and mental health. If you are struggling, please reach out to those around you for help. Some tips on how to do this include:

Share the Load Understand that it is okay to ask for help. Work colleagues may be able to step in and support you with the work you are doing. Sometimes we can be too proud to ask for help to our detriment. *Tip: We can get trapped into thinking that our colleagues will be unhappy with us if we ask for help. Asking for help can give others a confidence boost and our worries are often unfounded.*

Speak With Your PhD Supervisor Being honest with your PhD Supervisor may result in a reduced workload for a while to help you recover. They are also in a unique position to help you prioritise.

Ask for Extensions If you are overwhelmed with the amount of work you must do, ask for extensions. Many extensions are not set in stone. To do this, honesty is needed, saying that you need more time.

Consider Taking a Break Stepping away from your research can bring you back refreshed and ready to tackle your research. Taking time away can also lead to increased creativity.

Change Something Up Not all of us can take vacation time away from our studies for several reasons. In this instance, changing your day-to-day tasks for a short while may help. For example, if you have been working on writing a manuscript and are finding writing tough, consider working on the figures for the paper instead.

Temporary Withdrawal Most PhD programs offer the ability to temporarily withdraw (medical withdrawal) from a PhD program to concentrate on getting better. *Note: This is usually unpaid. Dependent on the country you work in, you may be entitled to several weeks of sick leave.*

> I withdrew from my PhD for 6 months on medical leave. It gave me time to get better and readjust my perspective when it came to my PhD work. When I returned, I had the energy and mental clarity to succeed.—PhD Student 3

Managing burnout can also be made much more difficult if you do not have the support of your PhD Supervisor. This might mean that they continue to give you a huge workload irrespective of how you are feeling, which can lead to increased stress. In these situations, seeking out support from your PhD program manager, or another academic you trust in your department may be prudent. Remember, without you, there is no PhD, no research output, and no subsequent changing the world. Put yourself first.

4.11 Navigating Self-Care as a Part-Time PhD Student

Managing being a part-time student comes with unique challenges, particularly when you may be working another job around your PhD study, managing chronic illnesses and/or caring responsibilities. In this instance, small self-care activities may be the most beneficial, like scheduling in coffee breaks for downtime, as well as giving yourself an evening or afternoon off per week (whatever works best for you) to decompress. With PhD study as a part-time student often spread over many years, taking a break may also not seem like a possibility through fears of not completing your program, but it is important to remember that burnout may mean you are not doing your best work, and that taking some time to rest is okay.

ADVOCATING FOR BETTER: How Can Universities Help Students Prioritise Self-Care?

Self-care is often considered the personal responsibility of students to implement, but there are several ways in my opinion that institutions can support self-care routines:

1. **Provide dedicated time for self-care:** Finding the time to actually do self-care can be tough for PhD students so making sure that there is time set aside for them to prioritise their self-care is important. This must be reinforced to PhD Supervisors so that they make sure that students take the time that they need.
2. **Challenge the culture of overwork and presenteeism [32]:** Strive to have staff model healthy behaviours and consider making out of hours working the exception not the rule. Taking time off with illness rather than coming into the department should be the standard.
3. **Ensure a living wage and hardship funding:** Financial difficulties can hugely impact mental health. Help can be provided by making sure that PhD students are provided a living wage (monitoring funding as a function of inflation etc.) and that internships are not paid in "experience" (experience doesn't pay bills). Further, financial reimbursement must be quick when students have to pay upfront for study related costs such as conference travel. Better still is not having students foot these costs in the first place. Hardship funding should also be made for students that need it.
4. **Provide affordable access to healthcare:** Strains from poor access to healthcare can impact mental health. Universities should be providing free therapy/counselling services as well as access to medical advice. In addition to being financially accessible, these resources should be available in a timely manner.

Understanding that ensuring that students have access to support both physically and financially is imperative.

---

ing: a review. J Exp Psychol Appl 6(3):236–249
10. Sleep Foundation (2022) Sleep hygiene. https://www.sleepfoundation.org/sleep-hygiene. Accessed 13 Apr 2022
11. Roehrs T, Roth T (2008) Caffeine: sleep and daytime sleepiness. Sleep Med Rev 12(2):153–162
12. Vallance JK, Buman MP, Stevinson C, Lynch BM (2015) Associations of overall sedentary time and screen time with sleep outcomes. Am J Health Behav 39(1):62–67

13. Stothard ER, McHill AW, Depner CM, Birks BR, Moehlman TM, Ritchie HK, Guzzetti JR, Chinoy ED, LeBourgeois MK, Axelsson J, Wright KP Jr (2017) Circadian entrainment to the natural light-dark cycle across seasons and the weekend. Curr Biol 27(4):508–513

14. Sleep Foundation (2022) Bedtime routines for adults. https://www.sleepfoundation.org/sleep-hygiene/bedtime-routine-for-adults. Accessed 13 Apr 2022

15. Masento NA, Golightly M, Field DT, Butler LT, van Reekum CM (2014) Effects of hydration status on cognitive performance and mood. Br J Nutr 111(10):1841–1852

16. Burrows T, Goldman S, Pursey K, Lim R (2017) Is there an association between dietary intake and academic achievement: a systematic review. J Hum Nutr Diet 30(2):117–140

17. Lipson SK, Sonneville KR (2017) Eating disorder symptoms among undergraduate and graduate students at 12 U.S. colleges and universities. Eat Behav 24:81–88

18. Anglin RES, Samaan Z, Walter SD, McDonald SD (2013) Vitamin D deficiency and depression in adults: systematic review and meta-analysis. Br J Psychiatry 202:100–107

19. National Health Service (2020) Vitamin D. https://www.nhs.uk/conditions/vitamins-and-minerals/vitamin-d/. Accessed 1 Mar 2022

20. Rasberry CN, Lee SM, Robin L, Laris BA, Russell LA, Coyle KK, Nihiser AJ (2011) The association between school-based physical activity, including physical education, and academic performance: a systematic review of the literature. Prev Med 52:S10–S20

21. Ito S (2019) High-intensity interval training for health benefits and care of cardiac diseases - the key to an efficient exercise protocol. World J Cardiol 11(7):171–188

22. Soria KM, Horgos B, Jones-White D, and Chrikov I (2020) Undergraduate, graduate, and professional students' food insecurity during the COVID-19 pandemic. SERU Covid-19 Survey

23. Woolston C (2019) PhDs: the tortuous truth. Nature 575(7782):403–407

24. CAMHS Professionals (2022) Types of self-care everyone should be made aware of. https://camhsprofessionals.co.uk/2020/04/05/types-of-self-care-that-everyone-should-be-made-aware-of-%F0%9F%8C%8D/. Accessed 20 Jun 2022

25. Cranford JA, Eisenberg D, Serras AM (2009) Substance use behaviors, mental health problems, and use of mental health services in a probability sample of college students. Addict Behav 34(2):134–145

26. Alcoholics Anonymous (2022) Find a meeting. https://www.alcoholics-anonymous.org.uk/. Accessed 3 Jun 2022

27. Tawwab NG (2021) Set boundaries, find peace. Little Brown, London

28. Ray R (2021) Setting boundaries. Macmillan, Sydney

29. Giurge LM, Bohns VK (2021) You don't need to answer right away! Receivers overestimate how quickly senders expect responses to non-urgent work emails. Organ Behav Hum Decis Process 167:114–128

30. Kahill S (1988) Symptoms of professional burnout: a review of the empirical evidence. Can Psychol/Psychologie canadienne 29(3):284

31. Aronsson G, Theorell T, Grape T, Hammarström A, Hogstedt C, Marteinsdottir I, Skoog I, Träskman-Bendz L, Hall C (2017) A systematic review including meta-analysis of work environment and burnout symptoms. BMC Public Health 17(1):1–13

32. Kinman G, Wray S (2018) Presenteeism in academic employees—occupational and individual factors. Occup Med 68(1):46–50

5

Not Another Yoga Session: University Wellbeing Programs and Why They so Often Miss the Mark

There's perhaps nothing more disheartening as a PhD student than receiving yet another impersonal email about going to a yoga session, or attending a webinar on "How to eat well" hosted by our institutions. I remember one particular day, when I was struggling heavily with my mental health, a mental health support email came round with the same content I had seen only a few weeks prior, and I felt even more deflated.

Due to chronic underfunding of mental health services at universities, perhaps it is understandable that these programs do not meet the needs of PhD students, but I argue that there is a duty of care and responsibility from an institutional level to ensure the safety of their students.[1]

According to the 2019 Nature report, only 29% of PhD students said that the mental health services at their university were tailored and appropriate to the needs of PhD students, and as little as 1 in 3 said that the one-to-one mental health support available was at least "adequate" for their needs [1].

It is important to remember that these programs have to be intentionally broad, as it is difficult to know exactly what students will be going through (though as I will discuss later in the book there is a whole host of commonalities in the PhD experience that can lead to increased stress and potentially

---

(Trigger Warnings: discrimination, harassment)

---

[1] I want to take a moment to recognise that there are amazing individuals within university mental health services who are working towards change and doing their absolute best to keep you well during your PhD, and genuinely care about your welfare. These people are phenomenal and are often doing a superhuman amount of work within a restrictive and underfunded system.

affect mental health which could be focused on). It is therefore easier to focus on broader topics, but what this does is leads to the delivery often feeling impersonal. Undoubtedly a whole host of changes need to be made and a balance struck to make wellbeing programs fit for purpose.

I want to state before I do a deep dive on wellbeing programs that I have no issue with yoga, or mindfulness, or the principle of looking after your wellbeing. I would not be writing this book otherwise. I think they are incredibly important. Yoga and meditative practices help a whole host of people manage stress and are great self-care tools. What I do take issue with is in some cases wellbeing programs implying that if *you* just try harder *you* can fix your own mental illness and that it is your individual responsibility alone to fix it. In my opinion, this is like prescribing a band-aid to fix a broken bone. This approach is deep-rooted in the clinical psychology "deficit model" [2] of disability, which suggests that psychopathology is the result of dysfunction and distress, and this occurs due to some deficiency within the individual struggling. I argue that the real problem for most PhD students is actually the barriers they face from society, the environment they are working in, the attitudes towards mental health from those around them, and from university management itself. This is the disability social model when it comes to mental health support and provision [3]. Thankfully more and more university-wide approaches are moving away from the deficit model, and towards the social model.

5.1   Reactive Not Proactive

Historically, many universities have adopted a reactive approach to mental health support for students, waiting until an issue arises before intervention, then referring students to on-site wellbeing support and counselling services [4]. In recent years there has been a move towards providing more proactive approaches for student wellbeing, which has resulted in the development of mindfulness sessions, resilience training, peer support groups, and much more. In principle this is really useful, so how is it that programs designed for intervention so often seem to miss the mark? For me there are several reasons:

The Lack of Authenticity Often wellbeing programs are "one size fits all". They are generic, and often due to lack of funding, they have been adapted from undergraduate support services, and are not well tailored to the PhD experience. What results is that the wellbeing program feels disingenuous, serving as a box-ticking exercise rather than a resource to actually help students.

Not Acknowledging the Environmental Factors at Play From experience, wellbeing programs tend to focus on what the PhD student can do to look after themselves, but does not discuss the structural and systemic issues that PhD students may face during their research programs (more on this in later chapters).

> [It's] like just sticking on a plaster rather than actually addressing the underlying systemic issues that create a need for these courses in the first place. If someone's wellbeing is suffering, it's not because they're not being "mindful" or "resilient" enough.—PhD Student 4

No Opportunity for Feedback/Follow Up Wellbeing programs historically have not always been developed in collaboration with PhD students [5]. This can be further limited if there is no mechanism for feedback, resulting in a wellbeing program that is not fit for purpose. Increased focus on co-production of resources, as highlighted through the UK University Mental Health Charter, is driving change in this area, but is not realised globally [6].

Inexperienced Trainers Sometimes the people delivering the training have little experience of what a PhD program is actually like. This means that when asked specific questions they struggle to help PhD students with their queries and concerns.

Lack of Consideration for Cultural Differences Depending on the background of PhD students, speaking about mental health in a public forum may not be comfortable. Further, initiatives that are designed to help, may be challenging for some. For example, therapy dog visits may pose a challenge due to fear of dogs, or due to the fact that dogs are considered ritually unclean in some religions [7].

Inherent Ableism Often the advice for improving mental health is to get more physical exercise, and/or eat "better" food. These in principle are a good idea, but fail to account for individuals that cannot get outside to do physical exercise (for example having a disability or experiencing agoraphobia). Nor do they account for individuals that may have a complex relationship with food, with eating disorders common amongst the graduate student population. In my experience, typically no alternative wellbeing advice is given.

It is this combination of the blanket email, the lack of authenticity, and the focus on tackling issues which seem so far away from the day-to-day issues we are facing that can feel incredibly disingenuous. And, let's be frank, a visit from the therapy dogs on campus is nice, but isn't going to fix mental illness.

Another considerable challenge to these proactive approaches to mental health support is that they are often simply not embedded in the research culture of our institutions: they are seen as a "waste of time". As a PhD student, given time pressures, and cynicism from faculty around mental health support, wellness programs often get bad rapport. Thus it is super easy for us to withdraw from participating in wellbeing initiatives entirely. It's certainly what I ultimately ended up doing during my own PhD. Despite this, I am now going to spend the next few paragraphs advocating heavily for why you should *consider* attending them.

5.2   Trying Something New

It is not often we reflect on why these wellbeing programs in academia/universities exist in the first place. I've become somewhat cynical over the last few years, and often see them as universities ticking a box labelled "mental health" and calling their job done. And in many instances I have observed this to be the case. However, we need to look at what these wellbeing programs can do for us in spite of this. If we take a step back, what wellbeing programs are giving you are tools to look after your mental health and bolster your self-care. And just like any tool box there are tools that are going to be fit for purpose, and some that, quite frankly, aren't. Just like you wouldn't try to use a crowbar to sculpt a statue, not every wellbeing event you attend will work for you. If we reframe these wellbeing programs into how they *might* help you they can:

- **Provide you the opportunity to try different techniques and methods for improved wellbeing**. Knowing what you dislike can be as powerful as knowing what you do like when it comes to self-care.
- **Connect you with other individuals who may be in a similar situation.** There is huge power in having other people to speak to about how you are feeling and knowing that you aren't alone. Pay special attention to who attends from your cohort.
- **Provide you with specific time dedicated to your wellbeing.** These sessions are university approved time to explore mental health and wellbeing providing you with an opportunity to take a step back from your research and have a breather.
- **Put you in contact with individuals that genuinely care for your welfare.** Attending these sessions can provide you with the opportunity to meet people in university mental health services that can provide support and point you in the direction of resources that might help.

So, next time you see a wellbeing session on at your university know that just because a previous session was not helpful, it doesn't mean that a follow up one is not going to work. By taking an hour out of your day to meet like-minded individuals, as well as the other possible advantages above, it might just be worth it. Worst case, it might just end up leading to an open and frank conversation with your peers as (whilst perhaps it should not be the case) one of the benefits of wellbeing programs often being so bad, is discussing with your colleagues how awful they are, opening dialogue, and connecting through solidarity.

Another big barrier to attending wellbeing sessions (or taking time out of your day for your own self-care) can be finding the time to go. This can be made even harder if your PhD Supervisor does not believe mental health is important or that wellbeing programs are useful. *Tip: If you want to attend the sessions, remember that you have a right to attend university sessions and to look after your wellbeing.*

5.3   Building Resilience

> Resilience: the ability to maintain or regain mental health, despite experiencing adversity [8].

"Resilience" is a term that is bandied around a lot, and understandably so [9, 10]. Resilience is incredibly important because studying for a PhD is *tough*.

In the description of what resilience is, it is defined as an "ability". I like this because it highlights that we can learn resilience, hone our skill, and improve on it with time. For me personally, I find that resilience is best described with an analogy: that it is in fact a shelter that we build to protect ourselves from stormy weather. During our PhD that weather may well represent the challenges we have to navigate throughout the PhD process itself, as well as anything else life deems to throw at us. How robust our shelter is—whether it is a barely standing wooden shed, or more a stone castle with a protective moat—depends on whether we have been given the tools that are fit for purpose to build a sturdy shelter (self-care) and if we have a strong support network (friends, family and sympathetic colleagues) to help supply the mortar and strengthen it. It is important to note that not everyone starts on a level playing field either—privilege plays a role. Generational wealth, or access to healthcare can all make a huge difference, so when building that resilience up, others around you may have part of that shelter already built. This is important to understand when helping those around you too. They may benefit from your support and guidance.

So what can you do to bolster your own resilience?

Understand That Saying "Yes" to Something Is Saying "No" to Something Else Our energy and time is finite, and thus if we say yes to an opportunity it is necessary to acknowledge that if we take on something new when we are already at capacity, ultimately we are sacrificing something else [11, 12]. That could mean delivering on another project to a sub-standard level, or impacting our self-care, pushing us closer to burnout. *Tip: If possible, wait 24 hours before agreeing to do something new. This can allow you to truly understand the time commitment and if you have capacity.*

Learn to Accept Constructive Criticism Accepting criticism of your work can be really tough, particularly when you've put all your effort in to it. It is important to remember that most critique is designed to help you grow and improve (if you already knew how to be an academic you would have your PhD already!) [13]. It can help to focus on what the intent of the feedback is – Do you need to be more concise? Did you not read the literature in full? This is all learning and something to improve on next time. An important part of growth is taking this on board, and bouncing back. I also want to highlight that sometimes feedback is **not** constructive. This might include using capital letters to reiterate points, or being overly harsh. Recognising that the feedback is not constructive is important for your wellbeing. *Tip: Consider, are they critiquing your work, or are they critiquing you directly?*

Realise Your Worth Is Not Based on Your PhD We can be so tied up in our education that we think that our worth is entirely linked to our academic outputs. This is not the case. Find joy in hobbies and activities outside of work if you can. These can help counter when you may feel low during your PhD program.

Build a Support Network Finding peers and colleagues you can speak to can truly help to share the burden of your PhD program. Make sure to speak to your family and friends about what you are experiencing too. We can think that our family is so invested in us getting a PhD that we cannot speak ill of it, but I guarantee that those that love you care for your welfare more. *Tip: Find like-minded PhD students in university societies and sports teams, as well as online through social media.*

Understand That 'Failure' Is Part of the Process Research not going your way can be hard to reconcile with. 'Failure' is not a bad thing (I use the term failure loosely as I think with all failing comes learning which ultimately isn't failure at all) as it is only by trying new things that you can discover something new [14]. *Tip: Reframe failure as a learning opportunity.*

Seek Professional Support Sometimes building resilience requires specific tools to help us improve it. This is where professional help may come in. Whether it is professional coaching, or seeking counselling there are many ways you might seek support. *Tip: Most UK universities offer a set of therapy/ coaching sessions for free. Try asking your graduate school for more information. Check with your university medical centre and find out what they offer. In some countries you can access reduced fee/free counselling services if your university as a clinical psychology/counselling training centre for their students.*

Finally, building resilience takes time. We often need to be exposed to situations to then learn to adapt to them. For example, the first time we experience a paper being rejected it *hurts*. Of course it does! It is only natural given that we put all our time and effort into it. But with experience (after taking a moment to address how we feel) we can learn to look over the feedback we get, make changes, and bounce back. Usually what we end up with is better than the manuscript we first submitted.

5.4   The Darker Side of Resilience

There is a darker side of resilience [15, 16]. Fundamentally there are certain situations that individuals should not have to be resilient through. This includes systemic issues, like racism, sexism, harassment and bullying, that are rife throughout the academy (discussed in more detail in Chap. 8) [17–19]. No-one should be subject to this behaviour. This should not happen, and much needs to change. Individuals that are victim to these abhorrent behaviours are often hugely resilient because they are forced to be. If this is you right now, know that you deserve to be treated with dignity and respect, and the situation that you find yourself in is not your fault. Know it is also okay[2] to realise you have reached a point in time where you have no resilience left to give, and that you need to put yourself first and walk away. Prioritising your wellbeing is perhaps the biggest act of defiance.

Resilience is also an easy "fallback" option for universities to rely heavily on, because then the onus for being unwell then falls on you for not being resilient enough. It can make us feel guilty and inadequate, when in reality we should not be being mistreated in the first place. This is gaslighting. Yes,

---

[2] It is not okay that the situation that you find yourself in has led to you reaching breaking point and having no more resilience left to give, but it is okay to prioritise your wellbeing.

resilience is important, but not acknowledging clear systemic issues that can impact mental health can be damaging. More on this in Part III.

> I'm tired of being resilient. I have more resilience than most and it still doesn't feel like enough.—PhD Student 5

ADVOCATING FOR BETTER: What Can Universities Do to Improve PhD Student Wellbeing Programs?

With the amount of financial support being put into PhD mental wellbeing programs, universities must consider evaluating and collecting feedback on whether the wellbeing programs that they are running are actually catered for the PhD students they are providing for. If they are found to be ineffective, a holistic view must be taken to remodel student support. There are several key areas that universities can improve on in my opinion:

1. **Realistic, frank conversations about mental health management and mental health literacy [20]:** This includes hosting events and discussions on recognising the signs of mental health distress in yourself and those around you, self-care, and discussing lived experiences through panel discussions or similar.
2. **Involvement of academic staff in wellbeing discussions:** This enables staff to understand the specific strains that PhD students are experiencing, particularly when supervisors may be out of touch with what being on a PhD program is like. *Note: caution must be taken to create student-only spaces too.*
3. **Acknowledging systemic barriers:** The research culture and the role it plays in increasing stress on PhD students must be acknowledged, or there is risk of disenfranchising the very students that wellbeing programs are designed to help. It is important to realise that systemic issues are sector wide and not just specific to a particular institution, so acknowledging they exist are not going to put students off your university, but they may help them manage their mental health during the PhD process. This involves moving away from the deficit model towards the social model for mental health.
4. **Teach students about their rights and resources available to them:** This includes how to set boundaries, how to change supervisor, and how to file a complaint about misconduct. Transparency around sick leave, maternity leave, and vacation entitlement is also needed.
5. **Create a sustainable, frequent program:** Putting wellbeing at the core of the PhD program is essential. This means having a targeted wellbeing program with content that does not repeat too often. Making sure the program is frequent and visible also helps to cement the idea that mental wellness is a priority.

Finally, perhaps the most important of all is recognising that no matter what wellbeing services you provide as an institution, if systemic issues prevail, it is like providing a boat with a hole in it out at sea, with little more than a bucket to stop the sinking. A two-pronged approach is therefore needed, focusing not only on managing symptoms but also managing the cause of systemic issues. There is no short-term quick fix to this, but recognising that the institution can influence and change the research culture is a necessary first step.

References

1. Woolston C (2019) PhDs: the tortuous truth. Nature 575(7782):403–407
2. Wally Y (2009) Disability: beyond the medical model. The Lancet 374(9704):1793
3. Barnes C (2019) Understanding the social model of disability: past, present and future. In: Routledge handbook of disability studies. Routledge, Abingdon
4. Williams M, Coare P, Marvell R, Pollard E, Houghton AM, Anderson J (2015) Understanding provision for students with mental health problems and intensive support needs: Report to HEFCE by the Institute for Employment Studies (IES) and Researching Equity, Access and Partnership (REAP)
5. Priestley M, Broglia E, Hughes G, Spanner L (2022) Student perspectives on improving mental health support services at university. Couns Psychother Res 22(1)
6. Hughes G, Spanner L (2019) The university mental health charter. Student Minds, Leeds
7. Berglund J (2014) Princely companion or object of offense? The dog's ambiguous status in Islam. Soc Anim 22(6):545–559
8. Herrman H, Stewart DE, Diaz-Granados N, Berger EL, Jackson B, Yuen T (2011) What is resilience? Can J Psychiatry 56(5):258–265
9. Casey C, Harvey O, Taylor J, Knight F, Trenoweth S (2022) Exploring the well-being and resilience of postgraduate researchers. J Further High Educ:1–18
10. Brewer ML, Van Kessel G, Sanderson B, Naumann F, Lane M, Reubenson A, Carter A (2019) Resilience in higher education students: a scoping review. High Educ Res Dev 38(6):1105–1120
11. Hinton AO Jr, McReynolds MR, Martinez D, Shuler HD, Termini CM (2020) The power of saying no. EMBO Rep 21(7):e50918
12. Grzyb JE, Chandler R (2008) The nice factor: the art of saying no. Fusion, London
13. Grenny J (2019) How to be resilient in the face of harsh criticism. Harvard Business Review
14. Topalidou I (2018) Teach undergraduates that doing a PhD will require them to embrace failure. Nature
15. Mahdiani H, Ungar M (2021) The dark side of resilience. Advers Resil Sci 2(3):147–155
16. Britt TW, Shen W, Sinclair RR, Grossman MR, Klieger DM (2016) How much do we really know about employee resilience? Ind Organ Psychol 9(2):378–404
17. Gillberg C (2020) The significance of crashing past gatekeepers of knowledge: towards full participation of disabled scholars in ableist academic structures. In: Ableism in academia: theorising experiencies of disabilities and cronic illnesses in higher education. UCL Press, London

18. Begum N, Saini R (2019) Decolonising the curriculum. Polit Stud Rev 17(2):196–201
19. Gabriel D, Tate S (2017) Inside the ivory tower: narratives of women of colour surviving and thriving in British academia. Trentham, UCL IOE Press, London
20. Schueth A (2022) Reducing the stigma of academic mental health can save lives. Nat Rev Urol 19:129–130

6

"I'll Read It Later" and Other Lies We Tell Ourselves: Managing Expectations and Guilt

During your PhD it is possible to get so hung up on what you "should" be doing that you can end up being paralysed by procrastination and guilt. In this chapter, I will focus on some of the common thoughts you may have which might ultimately lead to you accidently self-sabotaging your mental wellbeing, and how you might tackle them.

6.1 Starting Out

When you embark on your PhD journey, whether you have come straight through education without stopping, or are returning to education, there is likely going to be a change of pace. Depending on your location and institution this can go either way: you may find yourself swamped with additional classes and coursework to do, or you may find yourself in a very open-ended research project with little formal structure. Managing this transition can be tough. It is more than okay (and expected) for you to ask questions and seek support from colleagues and your supervisor. There are several factors that may result in you feeling a little overwhelmed in your first few months of your PhD:

No Clear Monitoring Points Unlike during undergraduate study, where there are a lot of exams and coursework, there is typically much less quantitative measures of your progress during a PhD. This can result in not knowing if we are doing enough to succeed and can make us doubt our abilities. It is

Z. J. Ayres, *Managing your Mental Health during your PhD*,
https://doi.org/10.1007/978-3-031-14194-2_6

therefore essential if you feel like this to ask for feedback from your PhD Supervisor on your progress. *Tip: Receiving feedback can sometimes be hard to hear, but everyone has something they need to improve on. The likelihood is you are progressing as expected.*

> I lost all concept of whether I was doing a good job during my PhD. It made me so anxious that I wasn't doing well, even though I had won several poster and talk prizes for my work.—PhD Student 6

Peer Perceptions Being surrounded by peers that are just as intelligent as you can lead to impostor feelings (discussed in the next chapter) and feelings of inadequacy. You may have gone from being top of your undergraduate classes to being average in your PhD cohort (reminder: average is still outstanding), and this can be a shock. Or you might be returning to education and need some time to recalibrate. It is important to remember that no route to a PhD is exactly the same, and therefore you may have a different background to those around you, but it does not mean you are any less capable.

Not Knowing Where Resources Are Something as simple as not knowing where resources are in your department, from where the printer is to where you can find mental health support can add strain during the first few months of your PhD program.

Being Away From Your Support Network Often starting a PhD means moving to a new town or city, or even a new country. This means that your support network may be suddenly long distance which can be hard to manage. Making new friends in a new location can take time. It is worth noting that these should improve with time, as you find your feet. *Tip: Consider joining university societies to meet like-minded individuals, and/or signing up to social media, and meeting people online through community hashtags such as #AcademicTwitter or #AcademicChatter on Twitter.*

6.2   Changing the World

Starting a PhD, we are often hugely optimistic (and rightly so). We have a tendency to think that our research is going to change the world, or feel the pressure to discover something truly unique. In the words of a good friend, in reality, it is more like "I might create something that might help the person, that helps the person, that helps the person, that helps the person that ends up curing cancer". Even then, it might not. Research is a gamble, and sometimes research directions lead to dead ends. The takeaway from this is important—your contribution to your field is likely to be small or incremental (this is the nature of research nowadays, as a large portion of the fundamentals of the world around us have already been discovered), but that does not mean it is not significant. You may never see the true impact of the work you do.

What you do achieve during your PhD is huge personal and professional growth. You will leave your PhD program with skills in how to manage complex projects, supervise students, and have gained a range of research skills along the way.

There is also often a mismatch between what we think we will achieve and what we end up achieving. That is normal, but it can take time to come to terms with. In truth, pursuit of a doctorate will only be a very small part of your contributions to the world over the course of your lifetime. By acknowledging this, we can release some of the hold our PhD might have on us. Yes you want to do your best, but it is not, and never will be your only defining contribution. Your worth goes beyond your PhD.

6.3   Planning Your PhD

During a PhD, one of the requirements is usually to plan your PhD output over the next few months or even years (cue the Gannt chart or detailed bullet point list of what you are going to achieve). When our research does not go to plan, it can result in us internalising feelings of not planning well enough. However, frontier research (exploring the unknown) cannot ever be truly predicted. So even the best laid plans will need to adapt and change completely during the PhD process. This is normal.

When we start our PhD we can also think that our PhD Supervisor knows exactly how our research is going to pan out, because they have experience in the field. In reality, given it is entirely new research, they have a rough idea of what *might* 'work', but this still does not mean that your project definitely will. *Tip: It may seem obvious, but remember that your PhD Supervisor is human, and does not know all the answers either.*

When we write down our research plan we also tend to write them in a very linear, stepwise manner, yet progress is rarely linear [1, 2]. The learning process is happening throughout our research, and the direction we take can be influenced by new information at any given time. Further, we can experience setbacks such as broken equipment, lack of access to resources that we need, or even having a range of unexpected admin or teaching to do, that means that progress is slowed compared to where we expected to be.[1] There are a range of "How to get a PhD" guides that you may find useful for planning your research (please see the up to date list in the online resources accompanying this book).

If you remain unconvinced, remember that you can explicitly ask your PhD Supervisor about if you are progressing at the expected pace for your own calibration. Dependent on your country of study there are also often yearly way-point checks with your PhD committee, which is a good indicator of whether or not you are working as expected. By asking the question, it means you can course correct if needed, though the chances are you are progressing just fine.

6.4   You Are Entitled to (and Deserve) Breaks

The often nebulous, open-ended nature of PhD study can lead us to neglect taking breaks and vacations. Internally we can justify this as there is always "more work to be done" and just keep powering through, with fear that if we don't we will not complete our PhD. Yet a PhD is a long process and can span from 3 years all the way up to around 10 years to completion depending on whether you are full or part time and/or require extensions or periods of leave. Objectively, not taking any breaks during what is a huge portion of your life is not sustainable—you have to have downtime. Taking a break can result in you coming back refreshed, with renewed energy and creativity to do your PhD work, although justifying wanting a break so that you will be more productive is not necessary: rest is a right, it is not earned. Life is short, and a PhD is a long time to not see friends and family. My advice would be to take the opportunity to see those you care about when you can.[2] This can really help with mood and mental health management.

Sometimes we can feel nervous to ask to take time off in the first place. We can think that perhaps our supervisor will think less of us for doing so. In reality the chances are that the time off will be granted, no questions asked. *Tip: Planning out your year and booking vacation time in advance so that you a). make sure to take your full holiday allowance and b). provide plenty of warning to your supervisor, can be a great way to ensure that you get all the vacation time you need.*

---

[1] Every year I thought I had planned my PhD a bit better and had been more realistic with timings and what I could achieve, and yet every year without fail I got it "wrong".

[2] I appreciate this is not always possible financially or otherwise.

> I was worrying about asking my PhD Supervisor for time off to go on holiday. I had worked it up into something much bigger than it was, and the email that came back in response to my request simply said "okay".—PhD Student 7

In some situations it may be your supervisor who prevents you from taking vacation time, and pushing back against this can be tough. Most PhD programs come with vacation time built in as standard, so knowing your vacation entitlement and your rights can be used to challenge this. If you are still struggling to take time off, joining your university union or graduate association may help you understand your rights further and provide support. *Note: Taking time off for faith-based celebrations should be granted. If this is denied this could be considered discrimination.*

You may find that by taking time off you may experience comments from colleagues or your supervisor "joking" about you taking vacation time. For example: "Off again are you?" or "How are you going to get anything done?". These may be examples of microaggressions if the implication is that any time off would be detrimental. It is important to remember that you are entitled to take vacation time, and that others should not be using shame to try and force you not to go. There is plenty of time during a PhD program to complete an original body of work, whilst still taking reasonable vacation time.

You may also experience pressure and feelings of guilt if you are constantly observing peers working late into the night on week days and working over the weekends. It is important to remember that working 24/7 is not a requirement to be successful.[3] Managing your mental health and staying well may mean that you simply cannot work these long hours—and nor should you. It is more than possible to get a PhD (and a good one at that) not working routinely out of hours.

6.5 Becoming an Expert

We can put intense pressure on ourselves to know everything about our subject area straight away. In reality, becoming knowledgeable in your subject area will take time (even for practitioners returning to study). There can be incredible internalised pressure to know everything immediately and, quite simply, you are not going to. Even towards the end of your PhD, you will have

---

[3] In theory, more hours in may mean more output, but this is only true to a point. It was this "grind" mentality that lead to me directly to burnout, which was not productive in the slightest.

accumulated knowledge but be aware that there is a whole host of information you still don't know. This is normal.

Reading the literature is a way to improve background knowledge. However, the sheer amount of existing research papers can be overwhelming. What results is a spiral of "I should be reading" or a backlog of papers and tabs open on our computers that in reality we are never going to catch up on. Understanding and accepting that that pile of papers is likely to just keep building can help us come to terms with the fact we will never know everything.

6.6   First Time Failing

During undergraduate and master's programs, the work we explore (particularly in STEM subjects) is designed to work, and the outcome is already known. For example, synthesising acetaminophen is a known chemical procedure, so as long as the protocol is followed correctly, the experiment *will* work (although those of you who have done organic chemistry labs will know that even then sometimes science doesn't always go to plan). When we start doing a PhD this all changes. All of a sudden we are doing research without known outcomes. This has to be the case to be exploring something novel that has not been discovered yet, but it doesn't mean that when our work doesn't go to plan that it doesn't hurt. To succeed we have to manage our relationship with failure:

Understand Research Requires a Leap of Faith Understanding what works and what doesn't helps us build a picture of the world around us and drive towards new, creative ideas. To do this we have to push boundaries and test where they break.

Know that Failure Isn't Actually Failure at All When we try new things and fail, we learn valuable skills along the way, such as perseverance, and technical know-how.

You Might Discover Something Else When your research goes off-piste, it is in these moments that you may end up discovering something that neither you or your supervisor have actually thought about previously and may end up going in a different research direction than you intended.

It Is Not Your Fault Research is research and it always has the potential to go in undefined directions. This is not your fault.

It is also important to remember you are a student. You are not expected to know everything and get everything "right". There will be a learning curve and this is expected.

6.7 Be Grateful (or Else)

If you are struggling during your PhD program, we can often experience a form of "survivor guilt". We feel we should be grateful for where we are and for the opportunity we have and this can result in feelings of guilt when we resent the situation we find ourselves in. Whilst gratitude is a good skill to practice, you do not have to be grateful if you find yourself in an unmanageable situation. Abuse does not and should not be tolerated—you deserve better than that.

On a similar vein, we can often feel compelled to enjoy every aspect of our PhD program, because if we don't we are "being ungrateful". In reality, there are going to be parts of any bit of work that you do not enjoy as much as others, or even dislike with a passion. This doesn't mean you are not a good PhD student, or that you are a bad researcher, it simply means that you are human. For myself, I really struggled throughout my PhD to sit down and actually read papers. I found my mind wandering after short periods of time, and it was almost impossible for me to do more than five minutes of reading a day. This led me to be hard on myself: other people were enjoying reading papers, why wasn't I? Did this mean I wasn't cut out for a PhD? Later I have realised that it means that deep reading of literature isn't for me. This didn't stop me from getting my PhD. *Tip: Sometimes our perceptions of what a "good researcher" should look like can be far away from the truth, and we can hold ourselves to unrealistic standards.*

6.8 Productivity and Time Management

It is natural to want to get from A (starting your PhD) to B (getting your doctorate) as quickly as possible. With that often comes both internal and external pressure to be constantly "on" all the time, thinking about your PhD, reading, and working towards your end goal. For that reason we can often guilt ourselves with statements like "I should be working" even though we have other aspects of life we are juggling. In reality, no human can work 24/7, and it is perfectly okay to have downtime. Yet it is not only outside of work

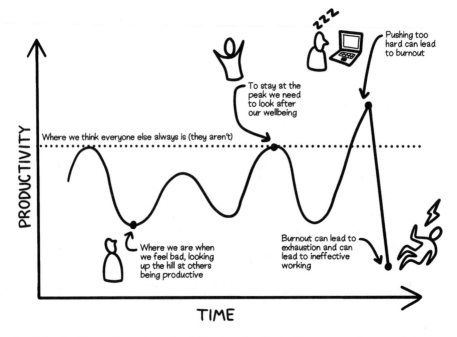

Fig. 6.1 An illustration of productivity showing that it has a waveform and changes over time

hours we can feel this way. We tend to have a perception that productive people are being productive all the time. This is simply not true. In fact productivity is a wave (Fig. 6.1).

Our concentration and productivity naturally oscillate. We will have periods of low productivity and high productivity, depending on our working style, wellbeing, motivation and other external factors. These periods could last hours, days or in extreme cases weeks. Again I will reiterate that particularly during a long-term project like a PhD this is normal.

Perhaps the most important of all—you do not have to be "productive" every day. You may find that one day all you end up doing is reading the same paper over and over again, and even then the information is not really "going in". The next day you may work 8 hours straight. Lean into this—listen to your body and what is working best for you on a particular day.

Comparing our unique working style with others can make us feel particularly rubbish. No project is the same, so comparison is like comparing apples with oranges—they are not comparable even though we might try. It is also important to note that we only see the output of other people when they are being the most productive. No-one in the working environment is going to tell you about the 3 hours they sat in front of their laptop screen failing to write more than two words whilst getting distracted by Reddit.[4] We may think that those around us, our colleagues, and our supervisor, do not have these moments, but I assure you they do.

Wellbeing plays a key role in productivity. If we get our self-care right, it means we are more likely to have the focus and energy we need to stay at peak performance for longer. So, investing in our mental health is investing in our output. Neglecting our wellbeing can also have other negative effects. If we keep pushing and pushing to be productive, paying little attention to our needs, ultimately we are likely to reach burnout. Burnout, a state of physical, emotional and mental exhaustion, can take a long time to recover from, during which time productivity is likely to be negligible. Establishing balance—pushing hard to be as productive as possible without going too far—is difficult. Unfortunately it is often a learning curve, finding out how far we can go, through trial and error.

Whilst productivity naturally oscillates, there are some tips and tricks I wish I had known to maintain productivity for longer, reduce the feelings of guilt, avoid self-sabotage, and ultimately improve mental wellbeing [3].

Divide Tasks Into Low and High Productivity Sets Given our ability to be productive can vary, assigning tasks into a more manageable set for low productivity moments (think file organisation, answering emails, building contacts on social media, reading literature)[5], and more difficult tasks that require more focus for when you are feeling more productive (e.g. writing/editing papers, creative thinking, data processing). This way, even in in moments where you are struggling with motivation, there are still some tasks you can do to be productive with the energy that you have.

Take a Break While it may seem counterproductive, taking a break and collecting your thoughts can actually lead to increased productivity. This can be as little as taking five minutes away to get a cup of coffee and refocus. Going for a walk can also help boost mood, whilst giving you the opportunity to think through the research challenges you are facing, with the added bonus of getting exercise. This still counts as work time.

Consider Using Productivity Tools There are a range of tried and tested productivity methods out there like the Pomodoro technique, which is designed to reduce self-interruptions by having a set time period (usually 25

---

[4] Okay you got me—this is me right now. You get the point.
[5] Note these are items I find easier to do in my "low productivity moments". That doesn't mean that they are necessarily suitable for you. Think about what tasks you find easier and designate them for when you are struggling accordingly.

minutes) where you intensely work, followed by a short break, then repeat [4]. Other options include online "Shut up and Write" community online sessions, designed to keep you accountable [5].

Remind Yourself of Why You Are Doing Your PhD A way to fight lack of motivation is to think back about why you embarked on the PhD process in the first place, as well was the main aims of your research project. Struggling to do that? Think about how you would speak to a room of people about your project. How would you make them excited about the work you are doing? *Tip: Keep these motivations on a post-it note in your workspace to remind yourself.*

Accept Time Pressure Might Be Your Motivator Everyone is different (personally I like to have any work done about a week before a deadline as I am an anxious person), but it may be that you procrastinate all the way up to a deadline. It is easy to feel bad about this, but I argue that sometimes we need these external motivators to drive us, so if you are delivering on the work just fine, even though you are working up to the last minute, if that works for you, it is *may* be okay to accept this and work with it not against it.

Understand "Golden Hours" We all have optimum working times. You may find that you don't work so well in the morning and are more productive in the afternoon or evening, or vice versa. A PhD often comes with the benefit of (at least some) flexibility so use this to your advantage. Work when is optimum for you if you can.

Realise That No-one Truly Works Efficiently for Long Time Periods When we are working a typical 8 hour work day, the amount of focused working time we actually do, on average is much less than this. The rest of the day is filled with chatting with colleagues, breaks, and small tasks [6]. Thus, if you are working from home, it is important to be realistic with your time—Did you get a solid few hours of work done? Great. No-one can be expected to sit there for 8 hours every single day working solidly without reaching burnout.

Use "This" or "That" Sometimes our PhD Supervisor's expectations on what we can achieve in a particular time frame are a long way from the reality of what we can deliver. In this scenario, saying "I can do this, at the expense of that" enables conversations about what work should be prioritised, whilst setting boundaries and highlighting that the volume of work is not achievable.

Have a "Scary Hour" We can often put off tasks that are a little bit scary to us, and they can weigh on us if left unaddressed. Scheduling a scary hour (or even a brave 5 minutes) each day where you face these tasks head on can really help [7].

Create a "Done" List With productivity sometimes we can dwell so much on what we need to do, we do not give credit to ourselves and what we have achieved. Creating a "done list" and adding to it as you go can be motivating.

With productivity it is also necessary to consider if you are being realistic with the number of tasks you have, and the amount of time you have to do them in. If you have too much work, having a frank conversation with your supervisor about delivery and expectations may be useful. Asking for extensions can also seem very daunting, but for the majority of cases you may get that extension granted. Remember: the worst that can happen is someone says no, and you are in the same position as when you started.

6.9 Prioritising

When we are overwhelmed with too many tasks and not enough time, taking a step back and taking some time to refocus can be incredibly useful. The Eisenhower matrix is a good tool to do this (Fig. 6.2) [8]. For me this helps me determine immediate actions and feel less overwhelmed. Through using a tool like this it may be possible to figure out prioritising your work on your own. It may also be beneficial to speak to your PhD Supervisor, or a postdoc to figure out what is the most urgent and important bit of work to do first. The most important thing is to realise that you cannot do everything all at once—it is not humanly possible. *Note: As time progresses through your PhD you will likely start to be able to prioritise with less reliance on input from others, as this is part of learning to be a researcher.*

> **Task**
>
> Write a to-do list of all items you need to do, then divide them into the Eisenhower Matrix categories on the next page (important and urgent, important but not urgent etc.). Then start on the task in the upper left corner of the matrix and work from there.

You may not be in a position to "delegate" to someone else to do the "urgent/unimportant" work. I certainly wasn't during my PhD. However, I liked to think of the "delegate box" as an opportunity to delegate work to myself on days where I have less mental capacity to do more complex work.

"To-do lists" can also be really helpful to manage your workload, though something I wish I had learned earlier in my PhD journey is to get comfortable with always having a to-do list in the background because the work is never done. Breaking down your tasks into more manageable chunks can help

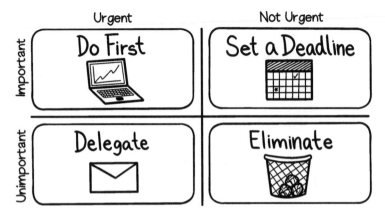

Fig. 6.2 Illustration of the Eisenhower Matrix

to feel a sense of achievement as you progress through your list. There is *always* more that could be done. Nonetheless, we have to take breaks, relax, and recuperate (without the guilt) to really innovate and do our best research. Work will wait. Your wellbeing won't.

ADVOCATING FOR BETTER: What Can Universities Do to Help PhD Students Manage Expectations and Guilt?

Transition from taught degrees, or from the world of work to a PhD can be a difficult one. Not understanding expectations can leave individuals feeling "lost at sea", thus, in my opinion, clear guidance as to what to expect during a PhD program is needed:

1. **Provide opportunities for feedback:** Given that doing a PhD can feel nebulous, providing clear feedback to students along the PhD process can be valuable. Though, care must be taken to ensure that this is guidance rather than rigid waypoints as each PhD experience is different.
2. **Allow for flexible working:** A 9–5 working time may not be suitable for PhD students, and some flexibility in being able to work at hours where productivity is higher (be this around caring responsibilities) or due to neurodiversity (and having periods of high intensity working followed by low intensity) is important.
3. **Give opportunities to learn time management skills:** Do not assume that PhD students are familiar with effective time management tools. Training should be provided, and a range of different productivity tools highlighted.
4. **Ensure and reinforce vacation time:** Rest is a right and should be treated as such. Vacation days should be accessible to all PhD students, and vacation day usage should be monitored to make sure no abuse of power is occurring (i.e. forcing students to work rather than take a much needed break).
5. **Consider mentoring programs:** Mentoring (whether from senior academics, or peer-to-peer) can help expectations to be managed and improve PhD student understanding of the PhD process.

References

1. Dunleavy P (2003) Authoring a PhD: how to plan, draft, write and finish a doctoral thesis or dissertation. Bloomsbury, London
2. Finn J (2005) Getting a PhD: an action plan to help manage your research, your supervisor and your project. Routledge, Abingdon
3. Kearns H, Gardiner M, Marshall K (2008) Innovation in PhD completion: the hardy shall succeed (and be happy!). High Educ Res Dev 27(1):77–89
4. Cirillo F (2018) The Pomodoro technique: the life-changing time-management system. Ebury, London
5. Mewburn I, Osborne L, Caldwell G (2014) Shut up & write! In: Writing groups for doctoral education and beyond: innovations in practice and theory. Routledge, London, pp 218–233
6. Kearns H (2019) 52 ways to stay well: during your PhD, Post-doc or research career. ThinkWell, Adelaide, Australia
7. Scott E (2022) This woman's 'scary hour' productivity hack could change your life. Metro
8. Crawford CM (2020) The 10 "C" s towards authentically supporting doctoral students: gracefully and successfully supporting doctoral students towards completing the capstone experience. In: Creating a framework for dissertation preparation: emerging research and opportunities. IGI Global, Hershey, PA

7

Why You Earned It: Fighting the Impostor

One of the biggest challenges you might face during your PhD is actually your own internal voice, telling you that you are not good enough, or don't deserve your place on your PhD program. This is called the Impostor Phenomenon or Impostor Syndrome. Feelings of being an impostor have been found to be frequently co-morbid with depression and anxiety [1].

The Impostor Phenomenon was first identified in the late 1970s, by psychologists Suzanne Imes and Pauline Clance in their ground-breaking work "The Impostor Phenomenon in High Achieving Women: Dynamics and Therapeutic Intervention" [2]. They found high incidence of feelings of "self-perceived intellectual phoniness" (feeling like a fraud) among participants in spite of clear evidence of external validation. Since then, it has been postulated that women experience impostor syndrome more than men, though recent reviews of the literature suggest that over half of the impostor phenomenon studies to date show no significant gender difference, meaning men are also likely to struggle [1].[1]

There has been a push in recent years to refer to feeling like an impostor the Impostor Phenomenon rather than Impostor Syndrome. This is because the use of "syndrome" is typically used to describe a long-term and pervasive medical condition and it is therefore incorrect to use this definition. Environmental factors also play a role, so the Impostor Phenomenon can be

---

(Trigger Warnings: discrimination, gaslighting)

---

[1] Note: there have been very little detailed studies on the effect of the Impostor Phenomenon on non-binary and gender diverse individuals. I want to acknowledge this. More research in this area is needed.

© The Author(s), under exclusive license to Springer Nature Switzerland AG 2022
Z. J. Ayres, *Managing your Mental Health during your PhD*,
https://doi.org/10.1007/978-3-031-14194-2_7

fueled by the environment we work in. For this reason, I will refer to feelings of not belonging throughout this book as "the Impostor Phenomenon".

The Impostor phenomenon is a paradox: other people believe in our abilities, yet we do not believe in ourselves. And yet, despite this, we listen to our inner voice telling us that we do not belong, over the views of other people who can objectively see our worth.

Elevated incidence of impostor feelings have also been observed in ethnic minority groups, particularly African American, Asian American and Latina/Latino university students. Several factors that increase psychological stress were identified, that fueled the impostor phenomenon, including being first generation (the first in the family to attend university), financial pressures, returning to study, and racial discrimination [3–5], indicating the problem is less about feeling like an impostor and more likely due to feeling actively unwelcome in academic spaces. Being part of any marginalised group within the academic setting (being LGBT+, having a disability (including mental illness), being a POC, or a woman etc.) can also lead to impostor feelings due to lack of visible role models [6].

The particularly tricky thing about managing feeling like an impostor is that you likely think that everyone else is struggling from the Impostor Phenomenon, but you are the **real** fraud [7].[2] Even now on reading this, you are likely thinking that I cannot see your unique situation, therefore you are the real impostor, and that I know nothing. For that reason I am going to use this chapter to highlight why you already deserve to be where you are, discuss how you definitely are not the odd one out (you really aren't), and how to fight these feelings when they happen.

It has been postulated that impostor feelings can also stem from being brought up in a highly achievements-focused environment [8]. Perhaps more praise was offered when you did well on a test, or drew a picture that was better than your peers. Perhaps you were always expected to achieve, high standards were non-negotiable, and there was no room given for you to be average at something, or just do hobbies because you enjoyed them rather than to excel [8]. The likelihood of this being the case as a PhD student is high, with on average only 1.1% of the world population (2% in the United States and

---

[2] It is also somewhat ironic me giving you advice to master the Impostor Phenomenon. I struggle with it heavily, and even now, am still working on my internal voice telling me I am not good enough. As I write this book, I wonder if it is actually just a load of rubbish and if I actually know what I am talking about. The fact that I hope that this is just the Impostor Phenomenon, not me actually being rubbish, is exactly the point—I think I am the odd one out and I am the real impostor. Maybe I am though? You get the point.

the United Kingdom) achieving a PhD [9]. This heavy focus on academic success is also why the Impostor Phenomenon often comes hand in hand with perfectionism (discussed in more detail later in this chapter).

To understand the Impostor Phenomenon, it is first necessary to understand some of the key aspects of a PhD program that may fuel these feelings. Work by Chakraverty (2020) explores some of the common themes that trigger the impostor phenomenon including: receiving recognition; receiving critique; comparing oneself with others; developing skills; application of new knowledge; and asking for help [10]. But first, we have to understand the value we bring to our research.

7.1 Understanding the Value You Bring

When surrounded by extremely talented peers, it can be easy to see the accomplishments of those around you and find it difficult to see what value you bring. And yet, all our life experiences (good and bad) are unique to us, and will shape what we contribute. Diversity is incredibly important when it comes to research; if we were all the same, there would be little innovation, and we would not address the full range of societal concerns through our research as we might not even be aware of certain issues that exist. This is illustrated by Fig. 7.1.

This diagram illustrates that we can be so focused on comparing ourselves with those around us and what they bring to the table, we often do not introspect and recognise the value we have. We can also often think that the only benefits from our background are those from our academic achievements too, but this is not the case. Growing up in a different neighbourhood, having different hobbies, having to be a carer for a family member etc., all give us unique perspectives and help with our research.[3] You never know where your skills might come in handy. It turns out hobbies are not just self-care, but can have practical use in our research too.

---

[3] In fact, I distinctly remember someone during my PhD using their painting skills to paint insulating epoxy onto (perhaps) the world's smallest diamond electrode to run their experiment, something no-one else had the knack for.

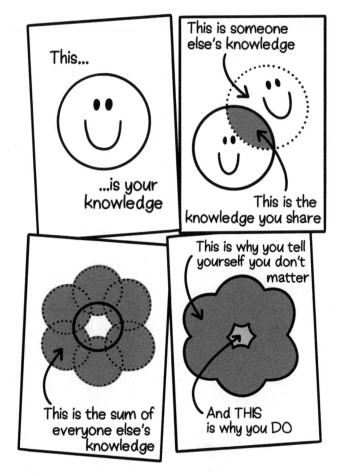

Fig. 7.1 An illustration on the impostor phenomenon and how we might look at the expertise of others in a positive light, but not give as much credit to our own expertise. Figure (redrawn to be in keeping with the book) with permission from Dr Heloise Stevance [11]

7.2   Receiving Recognition

Having your achievements recognised can be a double-edged sword when it comes to the impostor phenomenon. Our minds can use not getting our work recognised as evidence of us being "undeserving" of our PhD position. My mind used to say things like:

"I haven't been told I am doing a good job so I must not be good enough."

"My colleague won a poster prize and I didn't. I don't deserve to be here."

"I've not received any positive feedback recently from my PhD Supervisor so they must regret hiring me".

And yet, when I did get recognition, this fueled impostor feelings:

"They have got it wrong. I don't really know what I am doing."
"Someone else deserves this award—not me."

The first step in working towards managing these feelings is to realise that this is the Impostor Phenomenon talking, and challenging those thoughts.[4] A way to do this is to think "Would I have said that to a friend?" If not, it's likely your inner critic being too loud.

Next, is to reinforce to yourself as to why you are deserving of your PhD position in the first place. The fact that you were accepted for your PhD program) means that you have a proven track record of being able to think independently, conduct research, and have the background knowledge to succeed. That's right—you already have all the skills you need to complete your PhD. To be frank, if you were not capable, your PhD Supervisor would not take you on as a student because their time is valuable to them.

Task

An exercise you can do to remind yourself of why you deserve your PhD position is to write down on a piece of paper or sticky note:

- Your education and work experience up to this point.
- Five things you are proud of [12].
- Your five top skills.
- Any positive feedback you receive. By keeping this as a positive affirmation in your work space, it can act as a constant reminder of your ability [13].

Tip: If you struggle to write any of these objectively, ask a friend, colleague, or even your supervisor for help filling out these details.

Now looking at the recognition itself: during the PhD process (and academia in general) getting awards is highly competitive. Not receiving any awards does not mean you are not good enough. To be doing a PhD you are already exceptional (yes, really!). Of course, we would all like national and international recognition for our work, but in reality it is unlikely. *Tip: If you feel you need external validation ask your peers and/or your supervisor for feedback on your progress so far. This should happen as standard through milestone meetings.*

In the event you do receive an award, remember that there is typically a whole selection committee involved in making the decision on who wins an award. They have expertise in their field, and have been specially appointed to judge entries. The chances of them getting a decision wrong about awarding a prize are extraordinary low. Are you saying they don't know what they are talking about? I guarantee they have not got it wrong for you.

---

[4] Of course, calling out these thoughts and feelings is easier said than done. It takes time and practice to recognise them.

7.3   Receiving Critique

It is human nature to focus on the negative comments that we get. In some respects it is an evolutionary reaction, because it is ingrained to respond heavily and give more focus to situations that could "endanger" us. Unfortunately, critique can consolidate impostor feelings. Most of us remember a cruel or unnecessary comment and carry that with us, and forget all about the positive interactions that we had. This is why having that store of positive feedback is so important. It is also necessary to consider if the feedback is being given in earnest or not:

Consider the Intention Is it designed to help you improve your academic output and be successful? *Note: Sometimes, we can also read tone into written text, even if there is none.*

Decide if It Is Constructive or Destructive Particularly when we are struggling with impostor feelings, getting feedback that we are "doing a poor job" can fan the flames. Unfortunately sometimes critique can be given to intentionally knock us back. *Tip: Are the comments polite? Are the comments personal, not simply going through the work? If this is the case, they may be destructive.*

Ask for Clarification Sometimes comments can be "off the cuff", and yet they might stay with us for a while, long after the person said something to us. Asking "what do you mean by that?" so you can get more information may be useful.

Create an Action Plan If you have been given some genuine critique, actively consider what you could do to improve your skills and how you can get there. If you are unsure on your next steps, consider going back to the person that gave you the feedback and asking for help.

7.4   Comparing Yourself With Others

Easily done during a PhD, comparing your outputs with your peers can be almost impossible to avoid given how highly academia relies on metrics as a measure of success [14]. And yet, no two PhD's are exactly the same (they can't be else they would not be original research). This means that it is impossible to truly compare two PhD outputs. You may see people around you publishing lots, and wonder why you are not able to do the same. You may see someone's experiments working well, and be trying to get yours to work for the 20th time. This does not mean you are any less capable than them, just that you are on different research paths.

For me, as an undergraduate, I was top of my class and excelled at whatever I put my mind to before I started my PhD. Cut to being a PhD student, I was surrounded by people that were just as clever, if not smarter than me, and this came as a big shock, particularly as my self-worth up to that point had largely been pinned on my academic success. The often hyper-competitive nature of academia can exacerbate impostor feelings, as we can feel pitted against our peers. This is a problem with the research culture itself, where competitiveness is often rewarded over collaboration [15, 16].

One of the best bits of advice I can give you is to fight against competing with those around you and aim to collaborate instead.[5] Not only can this drastically improve your chances of publications (by joining forces and bringing together different skillsets) but also can help with your mental health, by having colleagues to share in the ups and downs of PhD study [17]. *Tip: the "successes" during a PhD can be few and far between, so finding joy in the success of others is a way to ride that high a little longer.*

7.5 Asking for Help

Being at the start of a learning journey can also be a shock: you may feel out of your depth, or not know where to start. This is where PhD Supervisors, senior PhD students and postdocs step in. It can be easily forgotten, but a PhD is a learning journey. If you knew everything, you would already have your PhD. You are not expected to know all the answers, or know detailed research methodology before you start. Given that everyone is so busy, you may feel like you are asking for a lot of help in the early days of your PhD, but this is entirely expected. You are not a burden.

Developing skills and application of knowledge can take even longer. You may have to ask to be shown how to run an experiment several times before it sinks in. Again, this is more than okay. You are learning. You also cannot be expected to know all of the literature in your field within a year, or even your whole PhD—there is simply not enough time in the day.

---

[5] I managed to get a fair few papers out during my PhD, which was in part luck, but also as I was good at identifying collaborations and choosing not to engage in competing.

7.6   Redefining Your Self-Worth

Starting a PhD, it's common (and normal) for the PhD to be a huge part of your life. A contributor to feeling like we don't belong is related to how we measure our self-worth and you may start to run into trouble if you tie your self-worth to only your academic success. As we discussed earlier, not everything "works" during a PhD and there are natural high and low moments. We can start to internalise feelings of "failure" when research doesn't go to plan, and consider it a personal failing of ours, rather than the research being difficult. Thoughts like "If someone else had been doing this they would have progressed much quicker" or "I don't deserve to be here as I keep failing" may start to creep in (which are absolutely not true but our brains are really good at lying to us). It is important to remember your contribution to the world around you (and your worth) is not based only on your studies. You are not required to prove your worth by getting that "experiment to work" or getting good qualitative data back, you already intrinsically bring value to your PhD program, simply by being present.

This is where having hobbies and an identity away from work is important: so that you have something to fall back on when your research is simply not working. Feeling good about ourselves through sports, art, or going to a pub quiz, watching Netflix etc., is important to decompress, as well as find our value in other things.

Our worth being pinned on our PhD studies can also trickle in to our social interactions. For example, introducing ourselves and focusing entirely on our PhD. Of course it is good to be proud of what you do, but it is not the only thing that defines you. *Tip: Look at your social media profiles and see how you define yourself. Does it just say "PhD Student"? Consider what else you could put in there as to what makes you, you.* This is important not only during your PhD but also afterwards.

Sometimes it might feel like an uphill battle to carve out time for a life outside of your PhD. Ensuring you are being productive with your working hours and having a clear cut-off for the end of your working day can help. The work will wait (see Sects. 4.9 "Setting Boundaries" and 6.8 "Productivity and Time Management" for more tips).

7.7   Perfectionism

The need to be infallible and excel at our jobs is deeply linked with impostor feelings. Striving for perfection may feel like the best way to deliver on our research goals, but it may in fact be detrimental to both our mental health and our work output. There of course can be positives to having perfectionist tendencies, such as attention to detail, but perfectionism can also be incredibly debilitating. Perfectionism can be broken down into two defined categories: excellence-seeking perfectionism and failure-avoidance perfectionism [18]. Both can be detrimental during the PhD process. Seeking "excellence" can lead to hours of wasted time, such as tightening up manuscripts when they are already good enough. Failure-avoidance perfectionism can lead to not taking any risks during the research process for fear of failure, which can inhibit learning and discovering new things. Perfectionism may take shape as [19]:

- Being hard on yourself and your outputs (more so than you would towards a friend).
- Worrying about what others think, including people-pleasing (putting the needs of others above your own).
- Procrastinating.
- Fear of trying new things, resulting in missed opportunities.
- Inability to relax during downtime.
- Constantly feeling not good enough.

If left unchecked these can be detrimental to your progress. Here's how you might go about challenging your inner perfectionist based on my experience:

Operate on the Principle of Sufficiency [20] As perfectionists, it is easy to fall into the trap of the "Principle of Ideality". This is where we are aiming to become the most "ideal" and most successful PhD student. In reality, this is unobtainable. It results in us pushing harder and harder, leading ultimately to burnout. Instead focusing on what is sufficient to get us through our PhD program is more sustainable. *Note: Most PhD programs are pass or fail, so it is okay to not be aiming for 100% at all times.*

Appreciate Your 80% Is Likely Many Others 100% If you are a perfectionist at heart, understanding that your 100% is likely overkill, and that a project doesn't need that level of commitment to be a success is important.

Perfect Is the Enemy of Done If you are focusing on everything being perfect, the chances are that you are going to take longer on each bit of work you need to do. This can be detrimental long term as it may result in you trading hours that could be used for self-care on finessing work that really did not need that extra effort. Further, when it comes to academic documents like papers and abstracts, your PhD Supervisor will likely provide feedback to help you improve on them anyway. They are not expecting you to get it perfect first time.

Test Boundaries One of the ways we can fight against our perfectionist nature is to actively deliver less on projects than what we would usually do. This can be very hard to start with, but you will quickly realise that less is in fact more. For example, setting a time limit on how much time you are going to spend working on a presentation, then working to that deadline.

7.8   Email 'Anxiety'

Experiencing impostor feelings can fuel concerns over sending emails, known as "email anxiety" [21]. This can result in spending large portions of time over the composition of an email, rewriting it and then being concerned about the reaction of the person that is going to receive it long after it is sent. This results in time lost that could be spent on research. Given that emailing is one of the most common forms of communication during a PhD, working towards managing these feelings is important:

Assign a Time of Day to Answering Emails If emails lead to increased stress and strain, dedicate a specific time of the day to managing your inbox. This way it is easier to contain feelings of worry and anxiety to during that time period.

Utilise an In-built Email Delay Most email systems have the ability to send emails on a delay timer. By sending emails with a delay, there is time to check over the email one last time and make sure you are happy before it sends.

Remove Your Work Email App from Your Phone You do not have to answer emails all day every day (and especially not in your evenings/personal time). Removing the email app from your phone means that it is much harder to access emails minimising time spent worrying about them outside of work.

Know People Won't Analyse the Content Like You Do [22] Most people will receive an email and give it a quick read over and that will be that. They will not be looking for hidden meaning in the email, and likely will not give it a second thought.[6]

Check It Is Polite The main thing when sending emails/requests is ensuring that they are polite. For example, have you used please and thank you? If so, the likelihood is that the email will be well-received.

Use Folders If you get overwhelmed by emails coming in, consider using a folder system so that emails that are read but require a later action go into a folder for you to address at a later date. This means that your inbox will not be entirely full of emails requiring actions when you log in.

7.9   Presentation Nerves

It is common to feel nervous before giving a talk on your research.[7] In fact, it is an indicator that you care about your research and that is a good thing—even if our bodies can overreact a little. Here are my top tips for navigating feeling anxious and/or nervous before and during delivering a talk:

- **Preparation is key:** Knowing your presentation content and being able to speak in detail about it is important, thus taking the time to prepare is necessary. If you do not have much time or notice, make sure to write down the key messages you want to deliver.
- **Have the first few sentences memorised:** Having the whole of your presentation memorised can work, but in some instances it can also make a presentation feel a touch stiff. If you have the first few sentences memorised you can get your presentation off to a good start and get into the flow of things, taking the pressure off.
- **Realise people are there because they want to be:** The people attending your talk are there to learn about your research. In short, they want you to do well. It can feel intimidating to stand in front of so many people but know they want you to succeed.
- **Remember you are the expert:** Although you may not feel like it at times, no-one knows more about your research than you do. If there is research

---

[6] I am terrible for this, and used to end up spending a lot of time on each email to make sure it was "perfect". In reality, as long as it is polite, there is no such thing as the perfect email.

[7] Even after having given over 50 (yes 50!) talks, I still get that sickening feeling in the pit of my stomach before speaking. In the past I have even taken my contact lenses out before giving a talk so I could not see the audience.

you do not quite understand yourself in your presentation it is okay to say that you are still interpreting the data, or omit that work entirely until you know more.

- **Find a "friendly" in the audience:**[8] Nearly always there is a smiling, nodding person in the audience. Find that person and look across at them from time to time during your talk. *Tip: There are often several people engaged around the room like this so you can look from one to the other to create a presence whilst you are talking.*
- **"That's a really interesting question":** Another common issue at conferences is a big-wig in the audience asking a question, which really isn't a question but a statement, which can make responding difficult. Having an answer ready to shut this behaviour down can be useful.

Finally, I'd like to add, sometimes our talks don't go quite as we would like, no matter how much we plan ahead. It is important to remember that you are learning and that also includes learning to deliver talks. Many of us are not naturally gifted at giving talks and it will take time. Further, we can be our own worst critics—the likelihood is that the people watching hardly noticed any moments you thought you "messed up". Be kind to yourself!

7.10 Fighting Back

So how might you start to combat that pesky Impostor Phenomenon?

Celebrate Little Wins as Well as the Big As PhD students we have a tendency to always delay gratification: "I published a paper, but I best start writing the next straight away". Celebrating the little wins as well as the big can help. This means getting an experiment to work, or even just getting out of bed. Our victories are different on different days.

Create a List of Your Achievements [12] Having a list of your achievements that you can look over in a low moment can help consolidate that you deserve to be where you are. *Tip: This could be as simple as scheduling in keeping your CV up to date in the event of a job coming your way, so that your CV is ready for when you need it.*

---

[8]Another thing to think about is—can you be the "friendly" for someone else? I try to do this, as I remember what it was like first starting out.

Speak to a Professional If the inner impostor voice is too loud and affecting you in your professional and/or personal life, speaking to a medical professional and seeking guidance is worthwhile. We can too often minimise the impact that feeling like an impostor has on us.

Call Out That Inner Voice Would you speak to a friend like that? If not, call that inner voice out actively. You deserve to be friends with yourself too.

Accept Recognition When receiving a compliment, it can be easy to be self-deprecating and laugh/joke about how we don't really deserve the recognition we are receiving. Next time you get given a compliment, try saying "thank you" instead.

Realise Perfectionism Is Not "High Standards" [23] We can get into a cycle of aiming for "perfect" and if we do not achieve this then we feel we are not good enough. If perfection is getting in the way of completing tasks, your perfectionism has become more a hindrance than a help.

Create a "Good Mail" Folder When you receive praise in an email, or kind communications, transferring them to a "good mail" folder to look back on when you are feeling low is a way to remind you of all the positive interactions that you have had and why you deserve to be where you are.

Now if you have read this chapter and do not experience the Impostor Phenomenon, there is nothing wrong with you—it is a great thing that you are confident in your abilities. You are not the impostor that actually doesn't feel like an impostor.

7.11 Discriminatory Gaslighting

> Gaslight (according to Oxford English Dictionary): To manipulate (a person) by psychological means into questioning their own sanity.

As a final thought in this chapter—is it truly the Impostor Phenomenon you are experiencing or is it something more sinister? Discriminatory gaslighting, where dominant social groups or individuals discriminate against and exclude marginalised groups, can amplify feelings of "not belonging".

Sometimes discrimination can be active, with targeted, cruel comments and be clear to see. Sometimes it can be much more subtle, leading to internalised feelings of doubt in one's own abilities. For example, there being few visible role models that look like you in your research department. For example, only 9% of Chemistry professors in the UK are women (this greatly affected me) [24]. Lack of representation like this can reinforce impostor feelings subconsciously. You may feel you do not belong but cannot understand why.

With the hyper-competition present within academia [25], it may also be that instead of being surrounded by supportive peers they see you as a threat and are putting you down to "elevate" themselves [26, 27]. This could take the form of "banter" mocking you for mistakes that you have made. Whilst this might seem friendly at first, or "just a laugh" it may be a form of manipulation to make you doubt your abilities. If you find yourself in this situation, try to surround yourself with people that lift you up not bring you down, and realise that it is their issue not yours. Of course this is easier said than done.

The culture of overwork can also consolidate impostor feelings, making care givers, including parents, feel as though they are not giving enough time to their work, and feel intense conflict between work and home life. Minority and historically marginalised groups may also feel they "do not belong" due to experiencing microaggressions and lack of representation. More on this in Chap. 8.

ADVOCATING FOR BETTER: What Can Universities Do to Help PhD Students Manage Impostor Feelings?

Managing internalised impostor feelings is not just an individual issue, but one that universities can work to improve, in my opinion, by:

1. **Provide Training**: If PhD students have not heard about the Impostor Phenomenon they may think that they are at fault or really do not belong. Holding specific seminars on the impostor phenomenon can help make sure students are informed.
2. **Not underestimating positive feedback:** Ensure that PhD students are getting positive feedback from PhD Supervisors, as its common for focus to be placed on the next research goal, rather than taking a moment to compliment the work that has been done. It is important to celebrate these wins.
3. **Provide opportunities for senior leaders to talk about feeling like an impostor:** There is one thing me talking about the Impostor Phenomenon in this book, but it is entirely different hearing that people in positions of power we respect and admire feel that way too. Putting on panel discussions to enable these discussions is useful to staff and students alike.
4. **Create networks:** Mentoring is incredibly valuable for PhD students, and can help build confidence and connections, as well as provide an opportunity to talk through feeling like an impostor with someone else in the field to get much needed perspective.
5. **Provide accessible healthcare:** Sometimes therapy is needed to really combat impostor feelings. This could be through talking therapy, Cognitive Behavioural Therapy (CBT), or similar.

References

1. Bravata DM, Watts SA, Keefer AL, Madhusudhan DK, Taylor KT, Clark DM, Nelson RS, Cokley KO, Hagg HK (2020) Prevalence, predictors, and treatment of impostor syndrome: a systematic review. J Gen Intern Med 35(4):1252–1275
2. Clance PR, Imes SA (1978) The imposter phenomenon in high achieving women: dynamics and therapeutic intervention. Psychother Theory Res Pract 15(3):241–247
3. Le L (2019) Unpacking the imposter syndrome and mental health as a person of color first generation college student within institutions of higher education. McNair Res J SJSU 15(5)
4. Holden CL, Wright LE, Herring AM, Sims PL (2021) Imposter syndrome among first- and continuing-generation college students: the roles of perfectionism and stress. J Coll Stud Ret 15210251211019379
5. Chapman A (2017) Using the assessment process to overcome imposter syndrome in mature students. J Further High Educ 41(2):112–119
6. Armstrong MJ, Shulman LM (2019) Tackling the imposter phenomenon to advance women in neurology. Neurol Clin Pract 9(2):155–159
7. Kearns H (2015) The imposter syndrome: why successful people often feel like frauds. ThinkWell, Adelaide, Australia
8. King JE, Cooley EL (1995) Achievement orientation and the impostor phenomenon among college students. Contemp Educ Psychol 20(3):304–312
9. Coldron AC (2021) How rare (or common) is it to have a PhD? https://www.findaphd.com/advice/blog/5403/how-rare-or-common-is-it-to-have-a-phd. Accessed 05 Mar 2022
10. Chakraverty D (2020) PhD student experiences with the impostor phenomenon in STEM. Int J Dr Stud 15(1):159–180
11. Stevance H (2022) Fuck impostor syndrome CC BY 4.0. https://www.hfstevance.com/graphics. Accessed 01 Nov 2021
12. Kearns H (2019) 52 Ways to stay well: during your PhD, post-doc or research career. ThinkWell, Adelaide, Australia
13. Boynton P (2020) Being Well in Academia: Ways to Feel Stronger, Safer and More Connected. Routledge, Abingdon
14. Fire M, Guestrin C (2019) Over-optimization of academic publishing metrics: observing Goodhart's law in action. GigaScience 8(6)
15. Hernaus T, Cerne M, Connelly C, Vokic NP, Škerlavaj M (2018) Evasive knowledge hiding in academia: when competitive individuals are asked to collaborate. J Knowl Manage 23(4):597–618
16. Moran H, Karlin L, Lauchlan E, Rappaport SJ, Bleasdale B, Wild L, Dorr J (2020) Understanding research culture: what researchers think about the culture they work in. Wellcome Trust, London, UK
17. Orford J (1992) Community psychology: theory and practice. Wiley, New Jersey

18. Harari D, Swider BW, Steed LB, Breidenthal AP (2018) Is perfect good? A meta-analysis of perfectionism in the workplace. J Appl Psychol 103(10):1121–1144
19. Frost RO, Marten P, Lahart C, Rosenblate R (1990) The dimensions of perfectionism. Cognit Ther Res 14(5):449–468
20. Axelsen D, Nielsen L (2015) Sufficiency as freedom from duress. J Polit Philos 23(4):406–426
21. Boyes A (2018) 3 Types of email anxiety and solutions. https://www.psychology-today.com/gb/blog/in-practice/201805/3-types-email-anxiety-and-solutions. Accessed 21 Jun 2022
22. Giurge LM, Bohns VK (2021) You don't need to answer right away! Receivers overestimate how quickly senders expect responses to non-urgent work emails. Organ Behav Hum Decis Process 167:114–128
23. Martin S (2019) Why you should strive for excellence, not perfection. https://psychcentral.com/blog/imperfect/2019/09/why-you-should-strive-for-excellence-not-perfection. Accessed 21 Jun 2022
24. Royal Society of Chemistry (2018) Breaking the barriers: women's retention and progression in the chemical sciences. Royal Society of Chemistry, London, UK
25. Edwards MA, Roy S (2017) Academic research in the 21st century: maintaining scientific integrity in a climate of perverse incentives and hypercompetition. Environ Eng Sci 34(1):51–61
26. Lashuel HA (2020) Mental health in academia: what about faculty? Elife 9:e54551
27. Täuber S, Mahmoudi M (2022) How bullying becomes a career tool. Nat Hum Behav 6(4):475–475

Part III

Environmental Stressors

8

Dismantling the Ivory Tower: Systemic Issues That Might Impact Your Mental Health

This Chapter is going to be a bit different than the others throughout this book. I am going to focus on the facts and figures (both quantitative and qualitative) around a range of discrimination and systemic issues that exist within academia so that you can grasp the scale of the problem. Honestly, writing this chapter was particularly tough to write, so I do not doubt for a moment that it will also be a tough read.

I will provide some details of how you can seek help at the end of the chapter, but "tips" and "tricks" will not be peppered throughout this Chapter. Why? Because navigating systemic racism, ableism, misogyny, bias and any other forms of discrimination is not something I can help you through with a statement or two. This does not mean that help is not out there, it just means that I want to acknowledge that it is a complex issue and not something that can be fixed by simply "changing your mindset".[1] Instead, a focus has been placed on providing some lived experience examples alongside statistics, so that you can start to understand some of the deep-set, challenging issues that many PhD students face, and know you are not alone. I see this as a start of a conversation that desperately needs to be had.

Perhaps one of the biggest lies we can be told is that our mental health struggles are entirely down to us "not being resilient enough", or that we are

---

(Trigger Warnings: suicidal ideation, depression, discrimination, anxiety, homophobia, racism, sexual harassment, bullying, classism, ageism, ableism)

---

[1] Not that those who experience discrimination are not superhumanly resilient, because they often have to be. But it shouldn't have to be this way.

the problem, not the environment we are working in. And yet, so often in academia it is the working environment that can make academia difficult to navigate [1–3]. I could not write this book with good conscience and not acknowledge the huge amount of systemic issues that can impact PhD mental health due to academic research culture. Many of these do not go away as we complete our PhD and stay present as we progress further in our academic journey, but many are also heavily compounded by power dynamics and the insecurity of doing a PhD.

With systemic issues, sometimes the biggest challenge can be recognising that they are impacting you in the first place. Not having noticed them is not a fault with you. Throughout my advocacy work, I have noted that these difficult topics often do not even get openly discussed by our institutions, or if they do, they get treated as behaviours so entrenched they are considered near impossible to fix.[2] Further, if these conversations are happening, often they occur behind closed doors, where senior leaders debate if these systemic issues even exist in the first place, as well as discuss how to fix them without appropriate representation there to provide much needed perspectives. In some cases, I have observed that these issues are considered to only affect a "minority" so appropriate time and budgets are not assigned to fix them. In other scenarios, people advocate for change for themselves, stopping once they have made the environment safer for their demographic, but then not stopping to lift others up too.

Whilst some universities are working towards change, in my opinion, there is a long way to go. Lack of exposure to these issues or not understanding the impact of them (both forms of privilege) also plays a role [4]. If our institutions do not tackle systemic issues, they risk driving out incredible individuals from academia, and the diverse perspectives that they have. You may be one of these individuals—it might feel like trying to wade through mud in order to survive and get your PhD—and I am truly sorry if this is the case. I want to remind you that you are **not** the problem.

I also want to emphasise that I am not saying that the onus for changing these behaviours is on you—it absolutely is not. The responsibility lies within our institutions, funding bodies and leaders in academia to drive for change from top down.

In reality whole books should probably be written on the topics covered in this chapter, and in some cases they have been (please see the resource list link at the back of this book). I have chosen to keep my coverage of each topic

---

[2] Just because something is hard to fix, doesn't mean our institutions shouldn't try.

brief, but I want to highlight that brevity does not indicate their importance. Each one of the areas discussed in this section need to be improved by our institutions, and whilst I cannot change that from here (at least not today) I hope that by reading about these you might at least start to feel less alone.[3] One of the biggest challenges as a PhD student can be realising that these systemic issues might be affecting your mental health, and how to articulate this to seek help. By writing about them in this chapter I hope to empower you.

It is also important for me to re-highlight that I am a cis-, white woman, from a working class family. Thus there are many systemic issues that I discuss in this chapter that do not intersect with my own identity. To this end, I thank those that I have spoken to that kindly discussed these topics with me and provided perspectives on the impact that these systemic issues might have for the purpose of the book. Further, if there is a section in this chapter that is missing, it is unintentional, but I, like everyone else, have my own unconscious biases and lack of exposure may mean I do not fully appreciate the scale of all problems that exist. Therefore if you do not find your particular struggles described in this chapter, that does not make what you are experiencing any less real or any less valid.

I also want to mention that for some aspects of discrimination that PhD students might face, there is little published on these areas intrinsically linking mental health concerns with these topics. Thus, in places throughout this chapter I have referenced PhD student data, and have also chosen to consider "early career researcher" to encompass and be synonymous to the PhD student experience.

Given the focus on lived experiences in this chapter, I also want to provide an additional trigger warning. Death by suicide, suicidal ideation, and discrimination based on a whole host of (what should be) protected characteristics are discussed. This makes for heavy reading and an emotional journey at times. The aim of this book is to help protect and bolster your mental health, so if you feel you cannot continue to read this chapter, there is no shame in that. Protecting your mental health comes first and foremost. I also want to remind you that there is information on how to seek help and support in Chap. 12.

For those that claim that these systemic issues happen elsewhere in other industries, and not just inside the academy: yes they do. However, as discussed earlier on in this book, the power dynamics involved with being a PhD student is heavily skewed so that PhD students have little power to change the situation they find themselves in. This can lead to abuse of power by the very

---

[3] Perhaps that is change after all.

people we should be able to trust. Further, a PhD is a time commitment of anywhere from approximately 3–10 years (and more in some cases like studying part-time). This is a long period of time, and once committed it can feel like a "waste" to leave part way through, even though as discussed in the final chapter of this book, sometimes leaving is the only valid option we have left. The decision to leave a toxic workplace is often harder when doing a PhD due a range of additional factors, such as having relocated, student loan debt, not wanting to disappoint those around us, and/or worrying about whether we would get the same opportunity again. For all of these reasons the research environment needs to be critically assessed to see if it is truly fit for purpose for everyone to thrive. Spoiler: It certainly isn't right now.

8.1   The Ivory Tower

Academia often gets referred to as an "Ivory Tower", which is defined in the English Dictionary as "a state of privileged seclusion or separation from the facts and practicalities of the real world" [5]. The important thing to note is that not only is academia exclusionary to those on the outside of academia, but there are a lot of exclusionary practices embedded *within* academia itself [6]. Many of these practices arise from historical lack of representation of marginalised groups within academia [7–9]. This can greatly impact mental health [10]. This leads me to the question: *What is the point of academia?*

I do not ask this to imply there is no point to academia or to be facetious. I ask it to make you stop and think for a moment. In an ideal world, at least from my perspective, academia serves society. It is designed to drive innovation to better humanity, inform public policy, educate and inspire future generations. And thus it follows, to be truly representative of society, we must have a diverse set of academics to truly solve the challenges of today and of tomorrow [11–13]. An Ivory Tower is the exact opposite of what we are aiming to achieve. The only way we start to dismantle this is by discussing that there is a problem in the first place. I certainly do not have all the answers on how we can address the wide breadth of research culture issues and discrimination that happen at our institutions, but I figure acknowledging them is a good place to start.

With all of the specific systemic issues I explore in this chapter, there is a theme that I believe runs throughout all of them: the sense of belonging, or more so, lack of belonging. When individuals feel "othered" this can ultimately impact mental health. In order to create a space where everyone can thrive, academia must aim to be inclusive and safe for all. Yet it so often is not. For each of the sections covered, it is clear that improvements need to be made at an institutional level.

8.2   Systemic Racism

Systemic racism is rife not just within academia but within our society as a whole, and is a significant challenge for people of colour (POC) to navigate [14, 15]. Spurred on by the #BlackLivesMatter Movement (originating on social media in 2013 by Garza, Collors and Tometi) change is happening, but it is slow, if not glacial within our academic settings [16]. The fact that systemic racism is rife within society, does not absolve academia from the responsibility to fix this either—supposedly progressive, universities should be leading change. Systemic racism at our institutions is not conjecture—the 2019/2020 Higher Education Statistics Agency (HESA) Staff report indicates that in the UK only ~0.7% of university professors are Black (155 out of 22,810) [17] which is in stark contrast to the UK population (~3.3% of the UK population is Black) [18]. Further, the UK Research and Innovation (UKRI) report "Detailed ethnicity analysis of funding applicants and awardees" shows that for funded doctoral studentships in 2019–20, 10% of students reported they were from an ethic minority background, which is significantly less than the HESA estimate of 18% minority ethnic students in postgraduate research, suggesting there is a systemic issue within funding bodies too [19].

Lack of talent retention further illustrates that there is a systemic racism issue within the academy, which is highlighted in the "Missing Elements: Racial and ethnic inequalities in the chemical sciences" 2022 Royal Society of Chemistry report showing that whilst 7.6% of STEM first degree entrants are Black (much higher than the UK population benchmark), only 1.7% academic staff identify as Black [20, 21]. It was also found in a Royal Society report that Black postgraduate students are the most likely to drop out of studying science (6.3%), compared to 4.4% Asian students and 3.8% for white students [22]. It is clear more must be done to prevent this happening. *So how might systemic racism impact your mental health as a PhD student?*

All of these statistics mean that there is less of a chance of "making it" in academia as an ethnic minority, which can weigh heavily. Lack of role models, and people to confide in who understand what you are going through can further exacerbate this. Further, exposure to both racism and microaggressions can be incredibly harmful, consolidating impostor feelings and feelings of not belonging.

An additional pressure to participate in diversity drives and in outreach initiatives to inspire the next generation can add strain, coined the "cultural taxation" [23]. Whilst these activities are valuable, the current academic system does not give equal standing to diversity, equity and inclusion work to other forms of academic currency like publications [24]. This can leave POC in a tough moral dilemma due to lack of recognition for such work [24].

Further, dependent on cultural norms, discussing mental health with family and friends may not be possible—it may simply not be a conversation that is considered acceptable due to stigma. This can be deeply entwined with religious beliefs, making it difficult to talk about complex feelings like suicidal ideation.

I was struggling to mingle at a conference so tucked myself at the back of the room. Someone stopped to ask me where they could get a program, and I realised that they didn't see me as a researcher, but as a member of the conference organisation staff.—PhD Student 8

A huge blow to my mental health was the death of my father during my program. I wanted to quit my program as a result, but I was pushed to finish by my family given the usual narrative of minorities needing to overcome these situations. As a result, I found myself to be the problem. I didn't want to be a burden to anyone and I felt I was a bad person, so I decided the only solution was to stop taking up space. The week of my PhD defence, I was extremely depressed and had major suicide ideation. [I felt] the temporary pain incurred in suicide would result in a lifetime of relief for everyone.—PhD Student 9

I have consistently wondered whether my race has played a role in varying capacities: from being told I had failed a research milestone because I did not recruit enough research participants during the pandemic (whereas a white woman the previous year had passed by recruiting even less individuals in non-pandemic times), to being unfairly singled out and asked difficult questions meant to embarrass me in front of others in the program. These experiences, in combination with seeing fellow POC cohort members face similar situations, has greatly impacted my mental health, to the extent that I had a major panic attack in year one of my studies. To this day, I do not recommend POC students apply to my program as racism remains a systemic problem.—PhD Student 10

8.3   Gender Discrimination

Sexism and gender discrimination is rife within academia, along with a range of conscious and unconscious biases, and not all of this happens behind closed doors [25, 26]. In fact, a recent example, which was branded "breathtakingly sexist" in an article in the US news outlet Time, was a public statement by Nobel Laureate Sir Tim Hunt at the 2015 World Conference of Science Journalists where he said: "Let me tell you about my trouble with girls ... three things happen when they are in the lab ... You fall in love with them, they fall in love with you and when you criticise them, they cry" [27]. Sir Hunt ultimately ended up issuing a formal apology and was forced to resign from an honorary professorship at University College London, "following the comments he made about women in science" [28, 29]. Further, a now retracted personal essay by Tomáš Hudlický (a prominent chemist) published in Angewandte Chemie in 2020, contained a diagram showing that "diversity of workforce" has a "negative influence" on organic chemistry, amongst several other controversial statements. This caused significant public backlash, including the resignation of 16 chemists from the journal's international advisory board, stating that "the disturbing act of Angewandte Chemie accepting and publishing an essay that promotes racist and sexist views, points to a larger problem wherein systems in the journal's publishing practices have suppressed ethnic and gender diversity" [30, 31].

What is clear, is that it is not just the personal opinions of the few that lead to barriers for women in academia, but that there is a range of systemic issues that women have to face in academia too. And as it stands, academia is far from equitable. For example, women hold 28% of professorships in the UK, despite women representing 46% of academic staff, and women making up ~half of the world population [17]. Thus, women are drastically under-represented in senior leadership roles. This so-called "leaky pipeline" where there is a significant attrition of women from academia, is the particularly prevalent in Science, Technology, Engineering and Mathematics (STEM). This can impact mental health through lack of role models, making it feel like success in academia is impossible. Further, there is a clear gender median pay gap of 13.7% for academic staff at universities in the UK, with women earning less than their male counterparts [32]. Further in the US, a report by Ohio University found that female faculty earn 11% less, equating to an annual loss of income of just over $26,000 USD [33]. As discussed in Chap. 10 there is also clear gender bias in academic publishing.

Academic workload allocation, particularly in terms of pastoral care duties and teaching also fall disproportionately on women [34]. This can affect the progression of women in academia, as any time away from doing research may impact measurable output, as pastoral care is often not considered "as significant" as research publications.

Perceived biases can also be incredibly difficult to navigate. For example, a white male professor in a recent survey stated: "When I say I have experienced and seen gender discrimination, it has always been against males. For example, we were directly told during a job search that we could not hire a white male, even though our relative representation of women and minorities is higher than average for our field. White males have long felt there is little likelihood of approval for sabbaticals or positive promotion decisions from the dean and upper administration" [35]. It can often be the belief that "positive discrimination" is giving the upper hand to a marginalised group, even though equity has not been reached in the first place. This may mean resistance/reluctance to change from those in senior positions.

When it comes to gender discrimination, non-binary and gender fluid individuals are often left out of the conversation, with focus on "women" and "men" in the research space. This includes when surveys are conducted to collect information on discrimination in the research space (inadvertently themselves being discriminatory), thus there is a need for more data collection to explore the mental health impact of PhD study for non-binary students.

So how might gender discrimination impact you as a PhD student? There are numerous ways that sexism and bias in research settings may present itself. A few examples include:

- Being spoken over in meetings.
- Someone presenting your idea as their own.
- Being expected to take on collegiate work/administrative duties over research work.
- Being told you received an award/got your PhD position as a "tick in the diversity box", rather than on merit.
- Experiencing microaggressions, including misogynistic jokes [36].

These can all impact mental health, adding to feelings of not belonging. Further, every day unconscious biases, for example, using masculine pronouns to describe a researcher: "The analyst should fill the volumetric flask up to the mark. He then should…", can add to the sense of "not belonging", and whilst it may seem insignificant to some, can weigh heavily, fueling impostor feelings. Having a supervisor that thinks that "no gender discrimination happens here" can make it difficult to get appropriate support.

My male lab mate during a talk expressed that women "Couldn't do extreme fieldwork." And that "Women couldn't use chainsaws." Because we couldn't lift and wield them. I was crushed. It was my first time being told to my face I "couldn't do" something because of my sex. It got in my head and whenever I failed or stumbled with my work I would hear those words repeated. I came very close to quitting. I would avoid going into the field with him because I felt like anything I didn't do up to his standards would be more proof that women weren't meant for this field."—PhD Student 11

During my PhD I had to disclose a medical condition because the diagnostic process and procedures meant missing class. They said, "Thank God. I thought you were going to say you're pregnant." Whenever I checked in later about missed classes they responded, "Okay, still not pregnant, great." I was experiencing hearing loss, vertigo, and confusion that was eventually diagnosed as Meniere's disease. All they seemed to care about was my womb status and if that would reduce my research productivity.—PhD Student 12

In my professional organisation, "gender minorities" has been used almost exclusively as synonymous with "women". Even though they seem interested in including non-binary folk, they tailor their work only to women and end up being exclusionary. I have also been struggling with what it means to "dress professionally", because more often than not it is interpreted to mean "dress masculinely", regardless of gender. Pant suits, no make-up or jewellery, etc. And so as someone who really rejects purely masculine (or feminine) representation, it has been hard to find a way to present myself professionally in an authentic way.—PhD Student 13

8.4   Sexual Harassment

Sexual harassment is defined by the United Kingdom Equality Act 2010 as "unwanted behaviour of a sexual nature which: violates your dignity, makes you feel intimidated, degraded or humiliated, and/or creates a hostile or offensive environment" [37]. This includes both physical advances as well as sexually charged jokes, inappropriate comments, gestures, the sending of sexual imagery, unwanted texts, emails, and social media contact.

Sexual harassment rates are high in the PhD community, with work by Rosenthal et al. (2016) finding that of 525 graduate students, 38% of women and 23% of men have experienced sexual harassment from faculty members, increasing to 58% and 38% respectively when looking at experiences of sexual harassment from other students [38]. Further 16% of graduate students reported experiencing sexual assault during their PhD studies.

Fieldwork, which is a requirement for several PhD programs, such as in the geosciences and archaeology among many others, has a long history of sexual harassment [39, 40]. Approximately 64% of respondents (70% women) have been exposed to sexual harassment during fieldwork, and 22% have been victims of sexual assault [41]. Similar findings have been found during work placements [42].

Despite sexual harassment being rife, support for victims is also not necessarily in place, with 48% of researchers in a 2020 CACTUS study stating they believe their institution does not have a comprehensive bullying and harassment policy [43–45].

So how might this impact your mental health as a PhD student? It is unsurprising that experiencing bullying and harassment can impact the mental health of victims. This includes affecting sleep and ability to focus; alongside feelings of hopelessness, anger, isolation, nervousness and depression [46]. Sexual harassment has also been linked with increased post-traumatic stress disorder symptoms [47]. Victims often feel less confident in their academic performance after an incident and may disengage from their academic studies [48].

The power dynamics of being a PhD student and experiencing sexual harassment from someone in a more senior position can make reporting an incident incredibly difficult. Unfortunately, this might make you feel like continuing with your PhD study in a particular research group/university is no longer a viable option for you.

> I was asked at a conference where I presenting a poster if the viewer (male) could take a photo of my poster. I said yes, as this is not uncommon practise, and I stepped out of the way. He then said "No, with you in it". I laughed and stayed standing away but he was being serious and didn't take the photo until I stepped back into the shot. I did this to avoid confrontation as people were waiting to pass etc. It was my first poster presentation and it severely knocked my confidence about the quality of my work. I considered whether was I getting attention for my scientific contribution or for other reasons.—PhD Student 14

> I'm a first year PhD student at a big university, and I was sexually assaulted last summer. My confidence and work output were severely affected. My supervisor was noticeably unhappy with my lack of progress. I didn't want to share about the assault, and only said I was going through severe anxiety. They said that "everyone has anxiety, you still need to do your job".—PhD Student 15

[I experienced] sexual harassment during my degree, and my lab mates reaction to it—"You didn't think he actually wanted to talk about your RESEARCH did you?"—made me withdrawal from interacting with more established scientists and potentially forming critical collaborations and finding mentors. I stop trusting my judgement and lost my sense of safety in my scientific community.—PhD Student 16

8.5 Bullying

Up to 43% of researchers have experienced bullying and harassment in the academy, while 61% have witnessed it [49]. This number increases considerably within the disabled research community, with 62% experiencing bullying and harassment [49]. Unfortunately 57% of PhD students do not feel they can discuss their situation without fear of personal repercussions [50].

Whilst we have talked in detail about bullying and harassment that may come from a PhD Supervisor (with ~60% of researchers attributing workplace bullying to their supervisors), bullying may also come from peers, flat mates, or other work colleagues [49].

So how might bullying impact you as a PhD student? There are numerous ways that bullying may present itself within the research setting, many of which are discussed in detail in Chap. 9. Examples include [51, 52]:

- Being called names that you find offensive or unkind.
- Exclusion from research meetings.
- Being shouted at or threatened.
- Being subject to microaggressions.
- Being unfairly criticised.

This may make you feel undervalued, excluded, and fearful of working within your research group. Experiencing bullying can also lead to feelings of isolation, depression, as well as anger.

I was bullied by our lab technician. She is known to pick certain people and hate them dearly and forever. I was unlucky enough to be one of these people. She seemed to spread stories about me so that other technicians regarded me with caution and mistrust as well. Whenever we met, she either ignored me or confronted me: Often, in lab meetings, she would immediately dismiss my ideas and talk down my experiments and interpretations. Whenever I made a mistake (which is normal!), they were made out to be the gravest and stupidest mistakes. I couldn't ask her for advice and help the same way my colleagues could.—PhD Student 17

As a PhD student I was harassed by a post-doctoral worker, who thought it was amusing to get in my way. I over-ran my PhD by over 4 months, costing me more than £10,000 in lost wages (Postdoc salary at the time), pension contributions and additional living costs because I was unable to start my Postdoctoral job in the US. It completely ruined the experience of being a PhD student and I lost out on at least one research publication. By the end I was at point of physical and mental collapse from having to work 15 hours a day.—PhD Student 18

When I went to my supervisor about being bullied she replied that I was making her life very difficult. I had to leave the room because she'd made me cry and I needed to take a break. When I returned she told me that "doing that" was very unprofessional and it wouldn't be acceptable in industry.—PhD Student 19

8.6   LGBT+ Discrimination

There is evidence to suggest that people that identify as part of the LGBT+ community have an increased risk of developing mental illness (1.5x higher than the general population) as well as increased risk of suicidal ideation [53]. This is postulated to be because, compared to those who identify as hetero-sexual, the LGBT+ community are more likely to experience discrimination due to their sexuality, alongside increased likelihood of being subjected to violence and abuse, and thus may be more likely to develop mood disorders such as anxiety and depression [54, 55].

In 2019 the Royal Society of Chemistry, Institute of Physics and Royal Astronomical Society reported 28% of lesbian, gay or bisexual respondents had at some point considered leaving their workplace due to discrimination; and 20% of transgender respondents considered leaving often [56].

A specific challenge for the LGBT+ community can be attending confer-ences and conducting field work, given that there are still several countries around the world where homosexuality is considered a crime [57]. This can result in lost opportunities and have a knock-on effect for future ones.

So how might LGBT+ discrimination impact your mental health as a PhD student? You may be victim to increased bullying and harassment during your studies. This can take many forms including name calling, sexual harassment, assault and exclusionary behaviour [58]. As a transgender or non-binary individual, you may be subjected to unintended (and intended) microaggres-sions misgendered through the use of incorrect pronouns [59].

"Deadnaming"—where a transgender person's name given at birth is used repeatedly, rather than there new chosen name is also bullying behaviour [59]. This can be inadvertently be reinforced by academic publishing practices that do not allow name changes of authors after publication, though thankfully this is changing [60]. This may make you feel isolated, particularly if there are not visible LGBT+ communities with your university and department.

> Routinely, when participating in diversity and inclusion initiatives I will hear someone say something to the tune of "sexuality does not matter". It does to me. It is part of who I am and if I am not accepted, it weighs on me and makes it harder to do my research.—PhD Student 21

> I heard a Professor say "LGB-well and the trans, whatever" when discussing the LGBT community, and it made me instantly feel othered, as well as question whether or not I was ever going to be safe and supported within my field.—PhD Student 20

> A large amount of my energy is spent towards worrying about my gender identity in grad school, and how it will hurt my mental health to be out, but also hurt my mental health to be closeted. There's no way to win as a non-binary person.—PhD Student 22

8.7   Being "First Generation"

Approximately one third of PhD students are "first generation" academics (where neither parent is university educated) [61]. With the exception of Asian doctoral recipients, the National Science Foundation 2020 "Doctoral Recipients from US Universities Report" found that first-generation PhD students are more likely to come from minority groups; with approximately half of Black, African American, American Indian, Alaska Native, Hispanic and Latino PhD students reporting neither parent having a bachelor's degree or higher (compared to ~ one third for White and Asian PhD students) [61].

Navigating academia as a first generation student can be tough. Work by Gardner and Holley (2011) highlights that lack of "cultural capital" first generation PhD students face, which is loosely defined as "lack of insider knowledge which is not taught in schools", making navigating a PhD challenging, as well as feeling isolated (both physically and mentally) from friends/family who do not understand the graduate school experience [62].

Further, research looking at tenure track faculty in the US found that of the 7204 faculty members surveyed, they were up to 25 times more likely to have a parent with a PhD than the general population, with about 22% of faculty having at least one parent who held a doctorate, highlighting that "generational wealth" and connections when navigating university systems is advantageous [63].

So how might being first generation impact your mental health as a PhD student? You may be the first in your family to attend university, or the first in your family to embark on a PhD. There is contention around whether the latter is truly "first generation" as if your parents went to university they at least understand a little about how the university system works, but even then, if none of your parents have done a PhD, embarking on a PhD can be difficult. There is often a whole "hidden agenda" to graduate school that you may not have any visibility to. This includes the need to publish, as well as networking with the right people to secure future jobs. It may come down to something as simple as not understanding PhD-related terminology which takes a while to learn. This ultimately means you may not be on the same playing field as others around you, and you may not have even realised this until now. This can impact mental health, particularly when comparing with others and their progress. You may feel like you do not "fit in", and/or struggle to relate to some of your peers.

> Not knowing a person that had been to university before me in family or friends, doing a PhD was difficult. I often felt like I didn't belong (still feel that now), and any questions I asked were stupid. Even my vocabulary was not up to scratch. I think that was the main issue for me, worrying about any questions I had or how I spoke, not knowing anything about how academia worked, what a grant is or even how the career path worked.—PhD Student 23

> As a first generation student, it's mind blowing when you find out about the hidden curriculum, and even more so when you realise that to many of your colleagues it isn't hidden at all. They had family to guide them, help them network early on, and who understands what it is they are doing.—PhD Student 24

Doing a PhD as an international, first-gen and state-educated student from a working-class background is already a lot. It means that you have to over-explain yourself because you have a different concept of the world as a whole, from being overly aware of privilege and calling it out, to stating what you consider the obvious in moments of injustice (e.g. supporting striking staff and unionising). This is draining on its own. If you add on top of that doing a PhD at a prestigious institution with very specific traditions, you end up being overly self-conscious of everything you do. It's honestly tiring to explain that I have lived a completely different life. I am not any less of a person just because I don't have these experiences.—PhD Student 25

8.8 Classism

Class discrimination (classism) is differential treatment, prejudice, or discrimination on the basis of (perceived) social class [64]. This is influenced by a range of socio-economic factors including wealth, income, education, occupation, and social network [64]. Unfortunately, classism (or elitism) is rife within academic settings [65–67].

Up to 60% of the UK general population self-identify as working class, yet, approximately 32% of students are from working class backgrounds, and even less at "Russell Group" (the UK equivalent of "Ivy League") universities [68, 69]. This is before the data is even disaggregated for PhD students. It has been found that those from working-class origins are "28% as likely to obtain a postgraduate degree when compared with their peers from more privileged origins" [70]. An example of where classism led to the death of a student is the case of a PhD student in the UK, who died by suicide, due to being mocked for "not being posh enough" [71].

So how might classism impact your mental health as a PhD student? This might appear in a simple question "Where did you go to school?" to bullying for sounding "common", having the wrong accent, or not feeling like you fit in in other ways. It also may present itself in terms of "professionalism", dictating what an academic looks like, in terms of clothing [65]. For example: if you don't have a tweed jacket and a leather satchel, perhaps you "aren't a real academic". Whilst this is of course nonsense, it can lead to a feeling of not belonging. Many of these feelings can be heavily internalised.

Historical class systems, like the caste system in India still impacts Indian PhD students to date, despite discrimination being banned on the basis of caste (called casteism). There have been a range of reports of PhD student suicides, which can be traced back to the students experiencing casteism, including discrimination, humiliation an exclusion, and not getting support from their universities [72, 73]. This is clearly a systemic issue.

> The final year of my PhD in Chicago I was thinking of doing some tutoring on the side to make a little more money. I told my dad, who is a professor, he said I should focus on finishing and then transferred a four-figure sum to my bank account. That obviously took any pressure off while clearly communicating the importance and feasibility of finishing. What a privilege! Throughout the PhD and afterwards, even when stressed with the end of contracts or visa renewals, I've always been able to rely on backing from my parents. I feel grateful for this, and know my whole career would have been much harder and more stressful without it.—PhD Student 26

> When I was studying for my PhD I experienced all sorts of classism and biases against me. Casual comments were frequently made and I was asked to say particular words because of my accent because "it was funny". All this low level stuff was just every day. One evening I was at a college dinner and someone complimented me on my watch. I said thanks and that it was a present from my parents for my 21st birthday. They laughed and said "Oh that's hardly an investment piece".—PhD Student 27

> Being from a working class background, I often felt left out of conversations or not in on the jokes (often about skiing holidays or simply being able to afford things). And I think a big thing is not knowing how to speak with peers and superiors. I've noticed people from higher socioeconomic backgrounds than me just effortlessly talk to the professors and network so well whereas I struggled to make conversation and feared networking! It's something I've worked on a lot and I feel I've made a lot of progress but I also definitely feel like I started on the back foot in this area.—PhD Student 28

8.9   Financial Concerns

Approximately, 55% of PhD students worry about their finances, and over half of PhD students report on having no exposure to formal financial education [74]. Further, underrepresented minority students are more likely to have to take out loans for graduate study, and 71% of all students who have taken out loans reporting being stressed by their situation [74]. Further, the 2020

SERU COVID survey of US graduate students revealed that 19% of graduate and professional students experienced food insecurity [75].

Financial concerns can also be aggravated by academic policies, for example, expecting PhD students to pay for travel to conferences out of pocket and get reimbursed later on. Universities and funding bodies must ensure that there is not just adequate support, but real, living wages given to PhD students.

Many graduate programs are paid at or around the poverty level, and with certain funding bodies paying a set stipend but not accounting for inflation, this can lead to financial concerns. An example of this is the Canada Graduate Scholarship ($35k CAD per year) for doctoral students, which has not changed since 2004 [76]. This means that whilst the cost of living has increased significantly the funding has not, making life more difficult, and resulting in living standards of PhD researchers dropping over time.

So how might financial concerns impact you as a PhD student? Studying for a PhD can be expensive, and even if you are receiving some sort of funding, PhD studentships are often funded poorly, and in some places are below the living wage. This can impact mental health due to worrying about paying rent and living expenses, as well as navigating reduced sleep due to having to work additional jobs to make ends meet. Now, navigating doing a PhD and part-time work should in theory be entirely manageable, but when combined with the so often encountered (unreasonable) expectations to be working 24/7 in academia, including working weekends it can make completing a PhD incredibly difficult. Financial concerns can also make prioritising self-care more difficult, for example, fresh ingredients to make meals are typically more expensive, and healthcare often comes with a cost, which may not be affordable.

> During my PhD I had to attend a conference in California. Between return flights UK-US, hotel costs and conference fees I was out of pocket to the tune of £2000. My university does not reimburse these costs until after you've attended the event, but you can't exactly pay for flights after you've already flown. I was out of pocket for over 8 months. I am lucky, I had savings and could just about afford the £2k. But I lost 8 months' worth of interest and stability on that money. Had an emergency happened, I would have ended up in debt.—PhD Student 29

> I don't know how PhD students are supposed to thrive and excel when they're worrying about surviving. I can't write well when I've not eaten all day. I can't sleep when I'm worrying about rent getting paid and if I can afford my bus ticket to get to the office. Wellbeing tips from my university about 'eating well to feel well' are so meaningless when I can't afford to spend more than 15p on noodles. It means only the privileged can succeed.—PhD Student 30

> The only months I wasn't worried was when I did problem classes and labs for the undergraduates because the extra money covered my rent. But that was only half the year and my supervisors (quite rightly to be fair) didn't want me demonstrating in the last year or so of my PhD so I could focus on my work. Fortunately I'm living with my mum and stepfather and so have little expenses but that just makes me feel worse, impacting my mental health, as I feel like I'm a burden on them.—PhD Student 31

8.10   Ableism, Disability and Neurodivergence

> Ableism (according to Oxford English Dictionary): Discrimination against people who are not able-bodied, or an assumption that it is necessary to cater only for able-bodied people.

Disability can be both visible and invisible [77]. 11.5% of postgraduate students have a disability in the UK, compared to only 3.9% of university staff declaring that they have underlying health conditions such as disability to their workplace [78]. This is in stark contrast to 16% of working age adults in the UK population declaring they have a disability. There are two possible explanations as to why there is this vast drop off in disability representation from postgraduate to staff: the first being as surviving in academia becomes more and more competitive moving up the academic ladder people are less likely to disclose their conditions due to fear of discrimination, or the second, that ableism within the academy drives these talented individuals out [79]. In reality, it is likely a combination of both. Brown and Leigh (2018) suggest that given stigma and ableism that exists, personal acceptance of disability may be lower [78].

Neurodivergent individuals may also experience ableism. The term neurodivergence encompasses a range of neurological conditions, including dyspraxia, dyslexia, attention deficit (hyperactivity) disorder (ADHD or ADD), Tourette syndrome, dyscalculia and autism [80]. It is important to note that neurodivergence may or may not be considered a disability, depending on various definitions, as well as if it impacts daily function.[4] Many of these

---

[4] Personally prefer to use the term disability as my mental illness can be disabling at times. I also choose to use "disabled" when it comes to discussing my mental illnesses, to fight my own internalised ableism around the word "disabled". This is of course, my own choice.

conditions require some form of learning accommodations, such as extra time to do assignments, and clarification of written instructions [81].

There is little data on the number of neurodivergent PhD student (or academic) experience. General workplace data suggests that over half of autistic individuals (60%) report their workplace behaving in a way that excludes neurodivergent colleagues [82]. Further, it has been reported that for students with an Autism Spectrum Disorder, many experience loneliness, which may contribute to dropping out from university [83]. In general students with disabilities are less likely to graduate.

So how might ableism affect you as a PhD student? Ableism can take many forms. You may happen across a professor that is unwilling to offer extensions to deadlines, even though you need an extension to complete the work. It may involve someone not believing you are struggling with mental illness because you "seem fine" due to invisible illness, because you do not fit their own internalised stereotype of what disabled people look like. Fear of disclosure may also impact your access to reasonable accommodations, due to concerns of how your PhD Supervisor/colleagues might treat you if they knew, due to stigma. You may also feel you have to put in 130% compared to others, just to get by, as well as find that even structures designed to help (like Disabled Student Allowance) involve so much paperwork and bureaucracy that they impede your progress [84].

If you are neurodivergent, you may notice a difference between your working style and what is considered "normative", for example, having periods of time with little productivity, followed by intense periods of hyperfocus. If your supervisor does not understand that and enable flexibility in your working patterns, this can be tough. You may also find that you need to ask for additional clarification to get tasks completed. "Masking" (hiding neurodivergent traits to "fit in") can also be incredibly tiring and increase the likelihood of burnout [85]. Not being understood can lead to increased feelings of isolation.

Navigating the PhD culture of overwork with chronic illness can also be incredibly difficult, particularly as long working hours are often lauded as an equivalent to a person's passion for their research (which is simply untrue). This may lead to you pushing through to do long hours at the expense of your health, or feeling like an impostor for having to take a step away from your research.

Further, your time to completion of a PhD may be extended if navigating chronic illness (which is not a bad thing, as taking care of yourself is priority number one), however, this may lead to increased financial stressors, which can in turn affect mental health. If you suspect you may be neurodivergent, speaking to a medical professional (if accessible) is a great place to start, or going to the graduate disability office for help.

> When I came back following 2 months of sick leave due to chronic pain and fatigue, my supervisor said that science doesn't work part-time. That statement still haunts me now.—PhD Student 32

> In one conversation, I light-heartedly told one of my supervisors that I always felt tired. She told me, sternly, that "You need to figure that out if you want to be a faculty member." She then proceeded to tell me how she felt tired in graduate school, but then realised she was sleeping too much. If only I slept less, then, my fatigue would go away! When I politely told her, "No, I think it's just my depression," she dismissed me. This is just one of many comments about my energy levels that I received in graduate school. I understand that people (probably) mean well, but, believe me, there is no quick fix for my disabilities.—PhD Student 33

> Throughout my PhD, I did various work for Equality, Diversity and Inclusion, and attended many department and college level committee meetings. Not once were neurodivergent minorities mentioned, let alone any possible support for them offered. Although I had reasonable adjustments from the university disability service that stated that I was allowed deadline extensions for assignments, I was met in person by the department disability officer and told that "We don't give those for PhD students as you're given enough warning in advance". Additionally, any help I was entitled to was completely inappropriate for me as it was all geared towards undergraduates and their needs which greatly differed from the support I needed to do my research.—PhD Student 34

8.11 Ageism

In the UK, a PhD student returning to study, after leaving education is often referred to as a "mature student", and ~ half of all PhD students are aged 30 or over [86]. Thus many people return to do a PhD later on in their lives, rather going straight through education to do a PhD.

Although improving, there are examples of embedded ageism within academia. For example, some awards are given to "early career researchers" based on age, not time spent working in a particular field.

Interactions with PhD Supervisors can also be complex, particularly if you have an established working style through experience of working elsewhere prior to doing your PhD, which can cause tension. This is usually due to power dynamics, and can be exacerbated if you are older than your PhD Supervisor.

So how might ageism affect you as a PhD student? Some of you may be returning to academia to do your PhD after an extended period working outside the academy, or some of you may be starting higher education at a later stage in life. There are several reasons that this may impact mental health. First, returning to study after a period away can be intimidating. It can take a bit of time re-adjusting to studying again. You may also find that careers support and advice for PhD students is tailored towards those individuals that have gone straight through academia without a break. Finding friends and colleagues to confide in, when not everyone is at the same life stage as you can also be difficult, particularly when it comes to mental health management. This can compound feelings of being an impostor, and that you don't belong.

> I started my PhD a few days before turning 32 years old. During my PhD, a white middle-aged professor—who I had just met during a professional dinner—told me that I was too old to be able to become a researcher. I was already not very comfortable with the fact that I was older than the typical PhD student, and I had a lot of doubt about what I am going to do after my PhD. These words of this professor piled on my anxiety.—PhD Student 35

> I'm an older returning student. I asked a professor I thought I had a good relationship with for a letter of recommendation. His response, "It's pretty unlikely someone at your stage in life would be successful in a PhD program. You have too many responsibilities outside of school".—PhD Student 36

> I was recently collaborating with a professor on a paper and noted they made a genuine (and assumably innocent) error in their statistical analysis. When I flagged this error and how correcting this changed outcomes, the professor without even reviewing my detailed comments said: "You are wrong, I've been researching this for longer than you've been alive".—PhD Student 37

8.12   Isolation and Culture Shock

Feeling isolated and lonely can occur at various times throughout PhD study. This might be due to doing long stints of research physically on your own, but it also might stem from others you care about not being able to understand the specific stressors you are experiencing in graduate school. This becomes a systemic issue particularly when there is little support given to PhD students who may be struggling, including not providing transition information to international students to help navigate a change in culture.

More than 50% of the UK full-time postgraduate population is made up of international students [87]. Moving to a new location, or new country can add additional strain, particularly with support networks no longer being accessible due to locale. Culture shock—feeling disorientation due to a change in way of life, culture, or set of attitudes (or all of these) can lead to feelings of isolation [88]. It is also worth noting that culture shock does not just occur due to travelling from one country to another, but can be experienced by people moving from the same country to a different state, or even someone experiencing a different socio-economic environment for the first time.

Social isolation has also been found to "contribute significantly" to students dropping out of their doctoral programs [89].

So how might this affect you as a PhD student? Being isolated from others may mean that you feel you do not have others to confide in. Feelings of loneliness may also contribute to a range of mental health issues, such as depression, alcohol abuse, sleep problems, and suicidal ideation [90].

If you are experiencing culture shock, you may feel homesick, as well as feeling lost [88]. You may find you have trouble concentrating and experience an increase in anxiety levels [91].

If you are an international student you may also be subject to bullying behaviour, such as being threatened to have your visa revoked, and/or be subjected to xenophobia, which can be isolating and impact mental health. You may also find asking for help difficult. Resources available to you are detailed in Chap. 12.

> After having lived in the UK for 5 years I had the most disappointing doorway question from my previous lead supervisor: "So, it's Christmas time. When are you going back home?" I my head I said "Right now". But then I said: "I do not know". After some time, you realise that for some people you will always be in the international student box no matter how hard you try to fit in this harsh environment and start your career.—PhD Student 38

> The writing-up period of my PhD was so very lonely. I felt that I had an almost impossible task to do, yet had no-one to turn to for support.—PhD Student 39

> Being away from my family and on a different time zone made it really difficult to speak to family frequently. At the start of my PhD there was a lot of good intentions around communicating frequently, but overtime this dropped off because life (and study) got in the way, and I felt very isolated.—PhD Student 40

8.13 A Comment on Intersectionality

Intersectionality, a term coined by Professor Kimberlé Crenshaw (1989), describes how different social identities such as race, gender, sexuality, class etc., contribute to the cumulative stress and discrimination that a person may experience [92]. Recently, work by Cech (2022) found that white able-bodied heterosexual men were uniquely privileged compared to 31 other intersectional groups in STEM, experiencing "more social inclusion, professional respect, and career opportunities, and having higher salaries" [93]. Further, the study found that this advantage was "especially pronounced when compared with the experiences of LGBTQ-identifying women of color, especially Black women, and for persons with disabilities across gender, race, and LGBTQ status [93]". This is not the first study to show this, with many studies showing disparities in pay, progress, and support, linking back to intersection with protected characteristics [94–97]. This shows that yet again that academia is not a meritocracy and that bias and discrimination weighs heavy within the academy.

If you are at the intersection of several of these identities, and relate to several of the sections discussed in this chapter, it may be even harder still for you to thrive in the research environment due to additional pressures and discrimination. This is where finding others to support you and share in what you are going through is important. This is discussed more in Chap. 12.

8.14   Changing the Research Culture

It is abundantly clear that more research is needed in these areas to truly explore the mental health impact of these systemic issues on PhD students, as whilst there are many studies on the impact of these issues on retention, there is limited literature linking them directly with PhD student mental health. I therefore conclude this chapter with a call to action to universities to explore these issues further.

I do want to highlight, however, that collecting data is only one step in the right direction. It is all too easy for institutions to fall back on "we need more data to make change", despite there being clear evidence that the research culture, fostered by the academy, impacts PhD mental health. Action needs to be taken. Further, surveys must be inclusive, and though often well-intentioned, may exclude individuals if not carefully considered.

8.15   In the Meantime, What Can You Do?

In this chapter, we have done a "whistle stop tour" through some of the systemic issues within academia you may be experiencing. After reading this section, I hope that the main takeaway message for you is that there may be a range of outside forces during your PhD program that may inadvertently effect your mental health. These are highly likely to be outside your control. They are also unfair, and should not be part of the academy. None of these behaviours are acceptable as a "rite of passage" for entry into the academy or "part of the job". They may make you feel undervalued and like you do not belong: but you absolutely do. Until real cultural change is realised though, it may be that you need to navigate these issues regardless to get your PhD. Some possible options for you going forward include:

Advocate for Your Needs It's all too easy for me to say this—is much harder to put into practice—but explaining to those around you the support that you need can be invaluable. Unfortunately this is a double-edged sword: self-advocacy can be draining and time consuming. You may find you simply do not have the capacity to advocate for what you need or have the words to describe what you need. It is worth remembering that by saying you are struggling with something to those around you opens up the opportunity for them to assist in finding solutions too.

Report Abusive and/or Inappropriate Behaviour If you feel able to (and please bear in mind it is absolutely understandable if you do not), use institutional reporting routes to report any incidences of bullying and/or harassing behaviour. If the behaviour is happening to you it is likely not a one off and is happening to others too. It is also important to remind you that if you do not feel safe reporting, you are not letting others down. You have to protect your own wellbeing first and foremost.

Educate Yourself The likelihood is that your identity does not intersect with all of the above. Thus, to help those around you, reading up on diversity topics to understand how you can be an ally can be useful. Do not be a bystander. *Tip: a good place to start is in the book "Being well in Academia" by Dr Petra Boynton, which as well as many other fantastic resources, has excellent information on how to be an **active** bystander* [98].

Find a Support Network One of the most important things to know is that even if you intersect with several of these areas, and feel alone because of this, there are people out there with similar experiences. They may not be at your institution—this is where the power of online spaces and communities really comes into play.

Know You Can Walk Away We will discuss this a bit later in the book, but know, nothing is worth your peace of mind, not even a PhD. If you are finding the environment you are working in toxic, it may be time to leave. It might not be the answer we want to hear, but know, there are safe, inclusive research groups out there, that treat PhD students with the respect and dignity they deserve. Most of all, know you are not alone in this. There is only so much a person can be expected to be resilient through. You deserve your PhD position, you bring value, and it is the academy that needs to change, not you.

8.16 Finding Light in a Dark Place

Whilst this chapter is full of the darker, scarier bits of academia, I want to take a moment to remind you that it is highly unlikely that all of these things are going to happen to you [98]. And even if they do, there is hope. In environments that make it difficult for us to thrive, it is often people around us—good, kind, and supportive individuals—that can really help us get through. This might look like a PhD Supervisor who is truly invested in your success, a colleague that understands the difficulties you are navigating and can offer a listening ear, or someone you connect with over social media, from across the globe that just so happens to "get it" too. In the final chapter we will talk a little more about finding and fostering connection, and communicating how you feel to ensure your success.

Further, there *are* universities working actively on research culture change, recognising their role, and trying to do better. There are people out there that will support and mentor you. There are people that care about you as a human being and want to see you succeed. This means that even if you are finding the systemic barriers at your current institution too high, you have options. Any institution would be lucky to have you.

ADVOCATING FOR BETTER: How Can Systemic Issues Be Improved for PhD Students by the Institution?

Addressing the research culture and environmental stressors that PhD students may face, in my opinion, is where universities can really make the biggest gains when it comes to improving the wellbeing of PhD students. This is because addressing environmental factors is a long-term solution, looking at the cause rather than fixing the effect of PhD student mental ill-health. There are many ways that these issues can be tackled, but, in my view, here is a starting point:

1. **Acknowledge that systemic issues exist**—It is only by recognising that a problem exists in the first place that we can work towards real, tangible change. This can also drastically improve the academic experience for PhD students, making them realise that it is not all in their head.
2. **Encourage open discussion and listen**—Creating open forums, or anonymous ways for members of your community to provide feedback on challenges and change that is needed, as well as then acting on that information, can help you tailor your approach for your department.
3. **Challenge the "this doesn't happen here" narrative**—It can be easy as senior leaders to believe that no bullying and harassment/racism or discrimination of any kind happens at our institutions, but the chances are it is absolutely happening, just behind closed doors. Not receiving any reports can be a sign that reporting systems need to be improved.
4. **Do not conflate gender equality with achieving diversity**—There has been much focus on improving (white) gender diversity within academia through initiatives such as Athena Swan, and things are slowly improving. This cannot be where diversity initiatives end. Other marginalised groups must be prioritised, and individuals that intersect multiple identities must be supported.
5. **Provide clear reporting routes**—Are there clear policies to report discrimination at your institution? Are they fit for purpose? Evaluating reporting routes and improving their visibility is important.
6. **Take complaints seriously**—There is nothing more disheartening than filing a complaint (which can take a huge emotional toll) for there to be no consequences for inappropriate behaviour. Universities must hold individuals accountable for their actions.

(continued)

(continued)

7. **Minimise paperwork**—Bureaucracy and a range of forms to fill out in order to get reasonable accommodations/temporary withdrawal/leave a PhD program can be ableist, and can add additional mental load on to PhD students that is not necessary. Streamlining necessary administrative documents, and ensuring everyone has access to reasonable accommodations is important.
8. **Create a collegiate community**—Focusing on collaboration not competition within the workplace can make a huge difference to the work environment. This must be supported by rewarding collaborative work.
9. **Reward and recognise DEI efforts**—Change-makers in departments must be recognised for their efforts to encourage further change. This means making sure that "success" is measured not only in paper publications, but also based on collegiate work.
10. **Ensure PhD students are financially supported**—A living wage can make a huge difference in whether or not a student successfully completes their PhD program. Further, ensuring that PhD students do not have to pay for conferences/travel out of pocket is essential. It is worth noting that international students may not be able to work additional jobs due to visa restrictions, which puts them in a precarious position. Hardship funds should be made available.
11. **Model the behaviour to be achieved**—Considering mental health holistically and looking at the strains and burdens on more senior academic staff is important, as PhD students are going to find it much harder to live values that maintain good work-life balance if those around them do not. This means addressing mental health support and provision, workloads and more at all levels in the academy.
12. **Signpost to resources**—Having the best support in the world means nothing if they are not visible and accessible for your PhD student cohorts. Making sure that frequent reminders about resources go out to both PhD students and staff is important to not only show where resources are, but also put mental health discussions on the agenda.

References

1. Carson L, Bartneck C, Voges K (2013) Over-competitiveness in academia: a literature review. Disrupt Sci Technol 1(4):183–190
2. Subbaraman N (2020) How# BlackInTheIvory put a spotlight on racism in academia. Nature 582(7812):327–328
3. Casad BJ, Franks JE, Garasky CE, Kittleman MM, Roesler AC, Hall DY, Petzel ZW (2021) Gender inequality in academia: problems and solutions for women faculty in STEM. J Neurosci Res 99(1):13–23
4. Johnston KV (2019) A dynamical systems description of privilege, power and leadership in academia. Nat Astron 3(12):1060–1066
5. Rawlins CM (2019) The ivory tower of academia and how mental health is often neglected. Future Sci OA 5(4):FSO392

6. Todd P, Bird D (2000) Gender and promotion in academia. Equal Opportunities International, Bingley, UK

7. Gillberg C (2020) The significance of crashing past gatekeepers of knowledge: towards full participation of disabled scholars in ableist academic structures. In: Ableism in academia: Theorising experiences of disabilities and chronic illnesses in higher education. UCL Press, London

8. Begum N, Saini R (2019) Decolonising the curriculum. Polit Stud Rev 17(2):196–201

9. Gabriel D, Tate SA (2017) Inside the ivory tower: narratives of women of colour surviving and thriving in British academia. ERIC, Columbus, OH

10. Limas JC, Corcoran LC, Baker AN, Cartaya AE, Ayres ZJ (2022) The impact of research culture on mental health & diversity in STEM, e202102957. Chemistry 28(9)

11. Medin DL, Lee CD (2012) Diversity makes better science. In: APS Observer

12. Kamerlin SCL (2020) When we increase diversity in academia, we all win. EMBO Rep 21(12):e51994

13. Hofstra B, Kulkarni VV, Munoz-Najar Galvez S, He B, Jurafsky D, McFarland DA (2020) The diversity–innovation paradox in science. Proc Natl Acad Sci USA 117(17):9284–9291

14. Feagin J (2013) Systemic racism: a theory of oppression. Routledge, Abingdon

15. Fiske ST, Massey DS (2021) Systemic racism: individuals and interactions, institutions and society. Cogn Res 6(82)

16. Garza, A. (2014) A herstory of the #BlackLivesMatter movement. https://the-feministwire.com/2014/10/blacklivesmatter-2/. Accessed 12 Jan 2022

17. HESA (2021) Higher education staff statistics: UK, 2019/20, Cheltenham

18. UK Government (2020) Population of England and Wales: ethnicity facts and figures

19. UKRI (2021) Detailed ethnicity analysis of funding applicants and awardees 2015-16 to 2019-20, London, UK

20. Royal Society of Chemistry (2022) Missing elements: racial and ethnic inequalities in the chemical sciences, Royal Society of Chemistry, UK

21. Royal Society of Chemistry (2020) Diversity data report, Royal Society of Chemistry, UK

22. Royal Society (2020) Ethnicity STEM data for students and academic staff in higher education 2007/08 to 2018/19, London, UK

23. Padilla AM (1994) Research news and comment: Ethnic minority scholars; research, and mentoring: current and future issues. Educ Res 23(4):24–27

24. Gewin V (2020) The time tax put on scientists of colour. Nature 583(7816):479–481

25. Savigny H (2014) Women, know your limits: cultural sexism in academia. Gend Educ 26(7):794–809

26. Cole K, Hassel H (2017) Surviving sexism in academia. Routledge, Abingdon

27. Greenberg A (2015) A Nobel scientist just made a breathtakingly sexist speech at international conference. Time

28. BBC News (2015) Sir Tim Hunt 'sorry' over 'trouble with girls' comment. BBC News

29. BBC News (2015) Sir Tim Hunt resigns from university role over girls comment. BBC News

30. Howes L (2020) Essay criticizing efforts to increase diversity in organic synthesis deleted after backlash from chemists. c&en

31. Krämer K (2020) Angewandte essay calling diversity in chemistry harmful decried as 'abhorrent' and 'egregious'. Chemistry World

32. Guibourg C (2019) Big university gender pay gap revealed. BBC News

33. Chen JJ, Crown D (2019) The gender pay gap in academia: evidence from the Ohio State University. Amer J Agric 101(5):1337–1352

34. Aiston SJ, Jung J (2015) Women academics and research productivity: an international comparison. Gend Educ 27(3):205–220

35. Woolston C (2021) Discrimination still plagues science. Nature 600(7887):177–179

36. Barthelemy RS, McCormick M, Henderson C (2016) Gender discrimination in physics and astronomy: graduate student experiences of sexism and gender microaggressions. Phys Rev Phys Educ Res 12(2):020119

37. UK Government (2010) The Equality act 2010. https://www.gov.uk/guidance/equality-act-2010-guidance. Accessed 21 Jun 2022

38. Rosenthal MN, Smidt AM, Freyd JJ (2016) Still second class: sexual harassment of graduate students. Psychol Women Q 40(3):364–377

39. Nash M (2021) National Antarctic Program responses to fieldwork sexual harassment. Antarct Sci 33(5):560–571

40. Voss BL (2021) Documenting cultures of harassment in archaeology: a review and analysis of quantitative and qualitative research studies. Am Antiq 86(2):1–17

41. Clancy KBH, Nelson RG, Rutherford JN, Hinde K (2014) Survey of academic field experiences (SAFE): trainees report harassment and assault. PloS One 9(7):e102172

42. Mennicke A, Kulkarni S, Ross T, Ferrante-Fusilli F, Valencia M, Meehan E, Crocker T (2021) Field note—Responding to the# MeToo era in social work: a policy for sexual harassment in field. J Soc Work Educ:1–9

43. O'Callaghan E, Shepp V, Kirkner A, and Lorenz K (2021) Sexual harassment in the academy: harnessing the growing labor movement in higher education to address sexual harassment against graduate workers. Violence Against Women https://doi.org/10.1177/10778012211035793

44. McCarry M, Jones C (2021) The equality paradox: sexual harassment and gender inequality in a UK university. J Gend Stud:1–13

45. Cerejo C, Awati M, Hayward A (2020) Joy and stress triggers: a global survey on mental health among researchers. CACTUS Foundation, Solapur

46. van Roosmalen E, McDaniel SA (1999) Sexual harassment in academia: a hazard to women's health. Women Health 28(2):33–54
47. Stockdale MS, Logan TK, Weston R (2009) Sexual harassment and posttraumatic stress disorder: damages beyond prior abuse. Law Hum Behav 33(5):405–418
48. Wolff JM, Rospenda KM, Colaneri AS (2017) Sexual harassment, psychological distress, and problematic drinking behavior among college students: an examination of reciprocal causal relations. J Sex Res 54(3):362–373
49. Moran H, Karlin L, Lauchlan E, Rappaport SJ, Bleasdale B, Wild L, Dorr J (2020) Understanding research culture: what researchers think about the culture they work in. Wellcome Trust, London, UK
50. Woolston C (2019) PhDs: the tortuous truth. Nature 575(7782):403–407
51. Moss SE, Mahmoudi M (2021) STEM the bullying: an empirical investigation of abusive supervision in academic science. EClinicalMedicine 40:101121
52. Mahmoudi M (2021) A brief guide to academic bullying. Jenny Stanford, Dubai
53. King M, Semlyen J, Tai SS, Killaspy H, Osborn D, Popelyuk D, Nazareth I (2008) A systematic review of mental disorder, suicide, and deliberate self harm in lesbian, gay and bisexual people. BMC Psychiatry 8(70):1–17
54. Chakraborty A, McManus S, Brugha TS, Bebbington P, King M (2011) Mental health of the non-heterosexual population of England. Br J Psychiatry 198(2):143–148
55. Dworkin SH, Yi H (2003) LGBT identity, violence, and social justice: the psychological is political. Int J Adv Couns 25(4):269–279
56. Dyer J, Townsend A, Kanani S, Matthews P, Palermo A, Farley S, Thorley C (2019) Exploring the workplace for LGBT+ physical scientists. Institute of Physics, Royal Society of Chemisty & Royal Astronomical Society, London, UK
57. Atchison CJ (2021) Challenges of fieldwork for LGBTQ+ scientists. Nat Hum Behav 5(11):1462–1462
58. Galupo MP, Resnick CA (2016) Experiences of LGBT microaggressions in the workplace: implications for policy. In: Sexual orientation and transgender issues in organizations. Springer, Berlin
59. Boustani K, Taylor KA (2020) Navigating LGBTQ+ discrimination in academia: where do we go from here? Biochemist 42(3):16–20
60. DePaul A (2021) Scientific publishers expedite name changes for authors. https://www.nature.com/articles/d41586-021-02014-7. Accessed 04 Jan 2022
61. National Science Foundation (2020) Doctorate recipients from U.S. universities. NSF, Alexandria, VA
62. Gardner SK, Holley KA (2011) "Those invisible barriers are real": the progression of first-generation students through doctoral education. Equity Excell Educ 44(1):77–92
63. Morgan A, LaBerge N, Larremore D, Galesic M, Brand JE, Clauset A (2021) Socioeconomic roots of academic faculty. SocArXiv

64. Class Action (2022) What is classism? https://classism.org/about-class/what-is-classism/. Accessed 04 Mar 2022
65. Crew T (2021) Navigating academia as a working-class academic. J Work-Class Stud 6(2):50–64
66. Langhout RD, Rosselli F, Feinstein J (2007) Assessing classism in academic settings. Rev High Educ 30(2):145–184
67. Rickett B, Morris A (2021) 'Mopping up tears in the academy'–working-class academics, belonging, and the necessity for emotional labour in UK academia. Discourse 42(1):87–101
68. Patrick B (2016) Most Britons regard themselves as working class, survey finds. The Guardian
69. DataBlog (2010) Does your social class decide if you go to university? Get the full list of colleges. The Guardian
70. Wakeling P, Laurison D (2017) Are postgraduate qualifications the 'new frontier of social mobility'? Br J Sociol 68(3):533–555
71. Lowe Y (2020) PhD student took her own life after classmates mocked her for not being 'posh enough', inquest hears. The Telegraph
72. Dhillon A (2017) 'A violence no autopsy can reveal': the deadly cost of India's campus prejudice. The Guardian
73. Maurya RK (2018) In their own voices: experiences of Dalit students in higher education institutions. Int J Multicult Educ 20(3):17–38
74. Denecke D, Feaster K, Okahana H, Allum J, Stone K (2016) Financial education: developing high impact programs for graduate and undergraduate students. Council of Graduate Schools, Washington, DC
75. Soria KM, Horgos B, Jones-White D, and Chrikov I (2020) Undergraduate, graduate, and professional students' food insecurity during the COVID-19 pandemic, SERU Covid-19 Survey
76. Khoo S (2021) How Canada short-changes its graduate students and postdocs. https://www.universityaffairs.ca/opinion/in-my-opinion/how-canada-short-changes-its-graduate-students-and-postdocs/. Accessed 04 Mar 2022
77. Davis AN (2005) Invisible disability. Ethics 116(1):153–213
78. Brown N, Leigh J (2018) Ableism in academia: where are the disabled and ill academics? Disabil Soc 33(6):985–989
79. Brewer G (2022) Disability in higher education: investigating identity, stigma and disclosure amongst disabled academics. McGraw-Hill Education
80. Clouder L, Karakus M, Cinotti A, Ferreyra MV, Fierros GA, Rojo P (2020) Neurodiversity in higher education: a narrative synthesis. High Educ 80(4):757–778
81. Brinckerhoff LC, Shaw SF, McGuire JM (1992) Promoting access, accommodations, and independence for college students with learning disabilities. J Learn Disabil 25(7):417–429
82. Management T.I.o.L (2020) Workplace neurodiversity: the power of difference

83. Van Hees V, Moyson T, Roeyers H (2015) Higher education experiences of students with autism spectrum disorder: challenges, benefits and support needs. J Autism Dev Disord 45(6):1673–1688

84. Hannam-Swain S (2018) The additional labour of a disabled PhD student. Disabil Soc 33(1):138–142

85. Sedgewick F, Hull L, Ellis H (2021) Autism and masking: how and why people do it, and the impact it can have. Jessica Kingsley, London

86. HESA (2022) Who's studying in HE? HESA, Cheltenham, UK

87. HESA (2022) Where do HE students come from? HESA, Cheltenham, UK

88. Hannigan TP (2007) Homesickness and acculturation stress in the international student. In: Psychological aspects of geographical moves: Homesickness and acculturation stress. Amsterdam University Press, Amsterdam, pp 63–72

89. Ali A, Kohun F (2009) Cultural influence on social isolation in doctoral programs and doctoral attrition - a case study. Inf Syst Educ J 7(64):1–7

90. Cantor G (2020) The loneliness of the long-distance (PhD) researcher. Psychodyn Pract 26(1):56–67

91. Hunley HA (2010) Students' functioning while studying abroad: the impact of psychological distress and loneliness. Int J Intercult Relat 34(4):386–392

92. Crenshaw K (1989) Demarginalizing the intersection of race and sex: a black feminist critique of antidiscrimination doctrine, feminist theory and antiracist politics. Univ Chic Leg Forum 1989(1):139–164

93. Cech EA (2022) The intersectional privilege of white able-bodied heterosexual men in STEM. Sci Adv 8(24):eabo1558

94. Scharrón-Del Río MR (2018) Intersectionality is not a choice: reflections of a queer scholar of color on teaching, writing, and belonging in LGBTQ studies and academia. J Homosex 67(3):294–304

95. Charleston LJ, Adserias RP, Lang NM, Jackson JFL (2014) Intersectionality and STEM: the role of race and gender in the academic pursuits of African American women in STEM. J Progr Policy Pract 2(3):273–293

96. Tao Y (2018) Earnings of academic scientists and engineers: intersectionality of gender and race/ethnicity effects. Am Behav Sci 62(5):625–644

97. Wolbring G, Lillywhite A (2021) Equity/equality, diversity, and inclusion (EDI) in universities: the case of disabled people. Societies 11(2):49

98. Boynton P (2020) Being well in academia: Ways to Feel Stronger, Safer and More Connected. Routledge, Abingdon

9

Perhaps It's Not You It's Them: PhD Student-Supervisor Relationships

If there is one thing that may truly make or break your PhD journey, it is the relationship you have with your PhD Supervisor.[1] Research has shown the interpersonal (professional) relationship between PhD students and their supervisors heavily influence the success of a PhD project, and is linked with progress and student satisfaction [1].

A good supervisor can lift you up when you are low, push you to be a better researcher, and continue to advocate for your success way beyond your PhD. Yet at the opposite end of the spectrum, a poor PhD Supervisor can bully you, gaslight you, and lead to a truly miserable few years of PhD study. In fact, in Nature's 2019 PhD student survey 24% of students when asked if they could start their graduate program over again, what they would do differently, said they would change their PhD Supervisor [2]. Again, I'd like to reiterate that I don't tell you these statistics to scare you, but to give you a better understanding of some of the issues you may face throughout your PhD journey.

It is incredibly important to understand early on both the impact a PhD Supervisor can have on your PhD studies, as well as that being a 'world-leading' academic does not necessarily equate to being a good mentor. Securing grants and getting published in high impact journals says nothing about someone's ability to look after the wellbeing of PhD students under their supervision. It is

---

(Trigger Warnings: bullying, harassment, sexual harassment)

---

[1] Depending on your country of study a PhD Supervisor may be called the Principal Investigator (PI) or you PhD Supervisor, or PhD Advisor. For the purpose of this chapter I will use "Supervisor", to mean the academic in charge of your PhD research.

© The Author(s), under exclusive license to Springer Nature Switzerland AG 2022
Z. J. Ayres, *Managing your Mental Health during your PhD*,
https://doi.org/10.1007/978-3-031-14194-2_9

possible to find someone that is greatly respected for their academic prowess and yet find them distinctly lacking in their mentorship capabilities.

For this chapter I will be focusing largely on the scenarios that the aforementioned 24% of graduate students experience—a toxic, unsupportive PhD Supervisor.[2] I choose to focus on the negative side of supervision and the impact it can have because it is only by discussing how this behaviour may impact you, that you may be able to recognise the behaviour you are being subjected to and work towards addressing it (through the parts you can control). Further, if you have a supportive supervisor who is a good mentor, you'll know just how important and helpful that is—imagine not having that support. That is what some PhD students experience. I truly hope that most of you reading fall into the other 76%, and that this chapter is largely irrelevant for you. One thing I will say is that whilst you may not be experiencing a difficult time with your PhD Supervisor, the supervisor-student relationship can vary very much from person to person. For example, whilst you might not be victim to bullying or harassment from your PhD Supervisor, it does not mean that your colleague that you sit next to isn't. Just a medieval knight, the champion of one person is armed and ready to take down another. Unfortunately bullying and harassment disproportionately affects people from historically marginalised communities, such as women, people of colour (POC), disabled people and members of the LBGTQ+ community, to name just a few [3]. This is one of the many reasons by poor supervision needs to be addressed at an institutional level, but often it is not.

9.1   Choosing Your Supervisor

Before you start your PhD, given the huge impact the PhD student-supervisor relationship will have on your success, it is important to chat to your supervisor before you start working with them.[3] Like with any job interview, just like you will be putting your best self forward during your first meeting, so will your supervisor. This means that it can be difficult (and even impossible) to truly gauge what they will be like as a supervisor.

One of the best bits of advice I can give is to speak to current and past members of your supervisor's research group and ask them what their experience was like. It helps to be specific with your questions. I would also recommend asking directly what the worst bits of the experience were, for example:

> Can you please give me 3 positive examples of working with [supervisor's name], and 3 negative examples?

---

[2] I count myself lucky every single day that I fell into the 76% category.
[3] If you did not get this memo before starting your PhD, please do not worry. It is common for first-generation students to not get this information ahead of time.

Asking directly means that you are more likely to get an answer.

Further, if mental health and wellbeing matter to you, perhaps due to past experiences with mental illness (so you know that you will need some support) or the fact that you want to thrive and not just survive your PhD journey, I would encourage you to directly ask your soon-to-be supervisor how they look after student wellbeing and what support is available at the university, as well as looking on your prospective universities website to see what services exist. Understandably we can be scared of asking our future supervisor these difficult questions. This is largely because there is still a lot of stigma associated with mental health and we often cannot fight the persistent feeling of "If I ask this will they not think I am capable?" or "Will they not take me as a student if I disclose my mental illness?". And it is true, they *may* think these things. But if they do, I have to ask, do you really want your next 3–10+ years of your life governed by someone that cares very little (if at all) about your welfare, or doesn't know the resources that are available to support you? Probably not. And, if they truly want to work with you, but have gaps in their knowledge on how best to support you, a good mentor works on this, to enable you to be the best version of you that you can be.

9.2   The Role of a PhD Supervisor

Across the world, there are different names that are used for the academic in charge of a PhD. For example, "Supervisor", "Advisor" and "Principal Investigator" are interchangeable, yet all meaning different things. In reality your PhD Supervisor has many different roles to play in order to deliver successful supervision (Table 9.1). The relevance of these roles is of course field dependent. For example, during a PhD in the sciences a PhD Supervisor may take on a "manager" role, but in the humanities, more self-led research may be expected.

On top of these, your PhD Supervisor is likely to have other responsibilities within your department and your research field. This may involve: lecturing; setting exams; marking coursework; being involved in a spin-out company; being representatives on international committees; diversity and inclusion work; being active practitioners in their field; pastoral care; external examinations; widening participation, among other things. This means that your PhD Supervisor is likely to be extremely busy. However, by agreeing to take you on as a PhD student, they also have committed to providing you the support and time that you need to have in order to be successful. You should never feel guilty for taking up your supervisor's time—they should have dedicated time to meet with you. Contact time should be formalised as part of the PhD process, meaning regular meetings take place at mutual convenience.

9.1 Different roles that a PhD Supervisor takes on during the PhD process, ed and expanded upon based on Vilkinas 1998 [4]

PhD supervisor job tasks	Description of support
Director	Contribute to research directions, providing ideas and expertise.
Teacher	Teach you how to navigate the academic process and teach you about relevant research techniques.
Facilitator	Provide access to equipment, funding, and professional contacts where needed.
Mediator	Assist in solving any minor disputes between research team colleagues.
Sponsor	Advocate for your success and put your name forward for opportunities.
Critic	Challenge you by providing constructive criticism of your work.
Manager	Track your progress, hold you accountable, and regularly provide feedback.
Developer	Check in on your wellbeing, and extend interest into who you are as a person (where appropriate).
Deliverer	Ensure you are delivering on research outputs and driving towards academic publications.
Examiner	Test your knowledge, run mock viva exams, and provide feedback on yearly progress reports.

9.3 Understanding What Makes a Supportive Supervisor

When we embark on our PhD journey we are often so focused on what we can bring to the table that we don't necessarily think about the skillsets that a supportive supervisor would have, and what we need from them to thrive. I'd therefore be remiss to not mention what a good supervisory experience looks like. In work by Rose et al. (2003), surveying several hundred PhD students only two traits were determined to be "extremely important" across the board: providing feedback, and communication [5]. This is not to say that other skills do not matter, but what it does show is that what an individual student's needs are, bar effective communication, are very different from person to person. For example, one PhD candidate may benefit greatly from a "hands-on" approach from the supervisor, whilst another may prefer a "hands-off" approach. If a supervisor approaches there role with a "one size fits all" mentality this is likely to cause problems.

It can be hard to assess if our supervisor is supportive based on the fact we likely do not know any different, so on the next page you will find a chart showing positive, supportive supervisor traits on the left, and negative, unsupportive actions on the right.

Task

Take a moment and think about your PhD Supervisor and your interactions so far, based on Fig. 9.1. How would you rate them on each attribute? Use the numbers out of 5 to give them a score, from 1 to 5 (5 being the most supportive). If your total number is close to the maximum of 40, your supervisor is likely doing a good job. If it is middling or lower, they may have room for improvement. Although not truly quantitative, this may give you some information as to whether there may be something amiss with the supervision you are receiving.

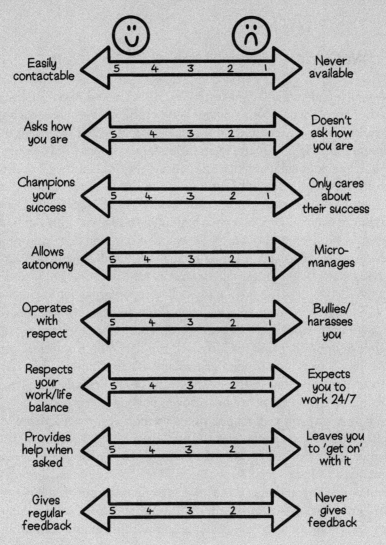

Fig. 9.1 Illustration showing PhD supervisor positive traits on the left, and negative traits on the right, with a sliding scale

I feel it is important to mention that supervisors are only human—they are never going to be perfect. They also may not know what they are doing "wrong" and will not be able to change that if they are not provided with feedback. There are however certain behaviours and mistreatment that you should never have to endure, like bullying and harassment and being forced to work 24/7. Understanding that you have the right to be treated with dignity and respect and that your supervisor is not infallible is essential for survival.

9.4   At Odds

Discussed by Vilkinas and Cartan (2006), the roles and responsibilities of a supervisor are often paradoxical to one another [6]. They explore that a supervisor must act in a 'developer' role, but also a 'deliverer' role. For a PhD Supervisor, this might be focusing on caring for the student and helping them cope with any personal issues that arise during the PhD journey, but also having to ensure that the student is productive and generating research outputs. This conflict is important to recognise as it helps to understand that your supervisor may not always have your best interests at heart. This can be tough to digest, as we often go into our PhD programs thinking that our supervisors will be our best advocates. Because of this conflict, I argue that your PhD Supervisor is not best positioned to be your *mentor*. Yes, some PhD Supervisors do a fantastic job of being mentors as well as supervisors, but I advise you to seek an independent mentor to help you throughout your PhD process [7]. This could be a senior PhD student within your research group, or another academic in or outside your research area. You may want to consider having a mentor that is working outside the academy. It's also important to note you can have more than one mentor, which can be particularly useful to get a wealth and range of experience to assist you in your endeavours.

So, how might you go about getting a mentor? It's worth looking around in your field and seeing who you admire. Then, simply, ask them. This can seem super scary, but I can guarantee that being asked to be a mentor is a huge compliment, and the worst they can do is say "no". It is also important to remember that if you do get a "no" this is likely to be due to the person you reached out to being overburdened, not because they don't want to help. And if they don't want to help, you really do not want them as a mentor anyway. The power is yours—ask!

9.5   The Flaw in the System

At present, many academics are not formally trained in mentoring [8]. In my opinion, there is still very much a "trial by fire" aspect to managing a research group, with you only getting training on the job [9]. Unfortunately, for the most part, the only people that are at risk of getting "burned" are the students that are the unbeknown guinea pigs. Academic promotions are typically achieved through publications and funding, not through successful mentorship, putting getting mentoring training much lower down the priority list, even for the most well-intentioned supervisors [10]. This is a systemic problem throughout academia that needs addressing, not only to improve the PhD student experience, but also to recognise some of the so-called "silent work" that often falls more onto female academics who are often deemed more approachable and end up dealing with pastoral issues more frequently [11, 12].

Further, there appears to be little opportunity for PhD students to give feedback to PhD Supervisors about their ability to mentor, and even when the lines of communication to give feedback are there (like having PhD student exit interviews for example) there is a huge power dynamic between the PhD Supervisor and the PhD researcher resulting in fear of repercussions [13]. By this I mean that all the power in the relationship resides with the PhD Supervisor. They determine how much support they provide you, what projects you get to work on, when you are ready to graduate, and your written references for any future jobs. So when the question: "How was I as a supervisor?" gets asked, the default is often to say everything was fine. This is understandable from the student's perspective—it's an act of self-preservation. This is a vicious circle as hearing that "all is fine" can ultimately reinforce to a PhD Supervisor that they are doing a great job. Couple that with having very little time for any self-improvement on their part (or really any motivation to do so, given how 'success' is measured in the academy) what results is a PhD Supervisor unintentionally (or intentionally) doing irrevocable harm to potential future researchers in their field. Sure, there are many instances where the supervision impacts students but is not so completely devastating that those students go on to quit their PhD programs, but even a small lack of support over time can lead to increased stress, all adding to the toll on your mental health.

There is also little accountability for being a bad mentor [14]. Harking back to the reward and promotions system in academia, supervision and more importantly the quality of that supervision rarely factors into tenure decisions, but the quantity of passes. There needs to be a lot of work done at an institutional level to enable ways for students to provide feedback on their supervisor and for student complaints to be dealt with discretion, as well as taken seriously. Things are improving though, with more emphasis on supervisors receiving training, as well as expectations for postgraduate training being formally outlined by funding bodies [15].

Recently, there have been several high profile cases where bullying and/or harassment has been reported, with institutions including research funding bodies taking action to remove funding and thus a large portion of power from academics that have been shown to abuse their position. There is hope.

9.6   Identifying Your Supervisor's Working Style

PhD Supervisors are as unique as the students they recruit, so any advice I can give on a supervisor's working style likely will not suit your PhD Supervisor perfectly, but I think it is an important reflective exercise—the more you can understand the impact of their management style, the more you can understand how their behaviour can affect your wellbeing. By understanding what might be going wrong, it enables better articulation of issues, and improved communication, all which can be channeled into "managing up" and managing your PhD Supervisor's behaviour. Should this responsibility fall to you? Probably not. But unfortunately this is often needed due to the lack of training given to supervisors.

Not exhaustive, there are a range of different supervisor "types" that fall into that 24% that you my come across, listed below [16]. A person may be one or many of these types combined. Under each type I have discussed possible ways you might manage this behaviour.

The Ghost   Barely ever present, with you having much less contact time than you need. They might use phrases like "it is up to you to explore this space" or "being thrown in the deep end is part of learning", which can make you feel like you are the problem, when in fact you are not getting enough guidance. They may be unavailable because they are overworked, or because they have tenure and do not really care about the success of their students.

How to manage this behaviour: Not having the appropriate amount of support can be difficult. In some instances it may be the case that your supervisor thinks you are capable and getting on just fine without guidance. To challenge this, explicitly ask for more contact time, and emphasise why that is important. If you still are not getting the support you need, look elsewhere. Is there a postdoctoral researcher that can help you? Or a colleague? You may also wish to actively seek an independent mentor.

The Laser Always watching you with laser precision. Barely gives you time to do any research and is constantly asking for updates which means you are constantly under pressure. This is more commonly known as being 'micro-managed'. You may struggle to actually get any work done due to the frequency of meetings and be made to feel inadequate for not producing more.

How to manage this behaviour: If you can, explain how the frequency of meetings is affecting your productivity and request that you have biweekly, or monthly check-ins as standard. Often this behaviour is about control, so it may help for you to send detailed plans of what you intend to do with your time before being asked.

The Scatterbrain They mean well, but their lack of organisation trickles over to you. This might mean that you end up with less contact time than you need (for example your meetings get pushed back), or you ending up doing a range of different activities including administrative tasks, and teaching additional classes that are not within your remit.

How to manage this behaviour: Setting boundaries can be tough, but it is important to remember you can say no to requests. For example, "Actually I have to focus on my research this week as we discussed" is a good way to remind your supervisor you have a PhD to complete. It is also worth considering—is doing these additional tasks adding to your skillsets which can go on your CV? If so, provided you still have time to do your research there may be benefits here.

The Paper Mill Sees you as a means to an end, and that is publications. They will drive you incredibly hard, often to exhaustion, and then even further. With the "publish or perish" mentality that is so pervasive in academia, one can easily see why some supervisors see their students as paper machines. They have little regard for you as a person.

How to manage this behaviour: This can be an incredibly difficult situation to manage. The temptation can be to just keep pushing on through, but for your wellbeing, breaks are important. Setting boundaries can start off small, for example saying "I cannot get the draft over to you on Sunday, it will

be in your inbox by end of day Monday". It is also important for you to recognise that your worth is not just in you citation success. Some people stick
this situation out because of the prestige of the research group they are working in, but bear in mind that you *can* leave. Nothing is worth sacrificing your
wellbeing over.

The Combatant They have taken a disliking to you and treat you worse than
a large portion of their research group and you are made to feel that you are
the problem. In reality you may not look or act like their "ideal" student, and
therefore they don't know how to manage you properly which can lead to bullying and abusive behaviour.

   How to manage this behaviour: If possible consider call out this behaviour in a public setting (but I also know how challenging and impossible this
might feel). The best course of action may be to report this behaviour formally
through the university. Often this combative behaviour is due to biases and/
or discrimination and should not be tolerated by the university.

The Optical Expert Recruits people for the optics. May have a group that
has good diversity but as soon as you get within the group you realise they
don't actually care about your welfare. They may use your ideas as theirs to
make sure that they always look "good" and ultimately only have their own
best interests at heart.

   How to manage this behaviour: Understand that they are likely to be a
poor mentor and seek a mentor elsewhere. It may be prudent to warn others
considering joining the group of the situation. If possible challenge the use of
your ideas as their own.

The Predator They know about the power dynamic that exists between PhD
Supervisor and student and use it. They know they control your "academic"
fate and use it against you. They may sexually harass, and/or force you to work
inhumane hours, and threaten to not give you a good reference when you
leave if you do not comply.

   How to manage this behaviour: This supervisor behaviour is in breach of
the code of conduct of your university and, if you feel able to, should be
reported. If going through formal routes of reporting is overwhelming, seek
support from friends or family to help you through the process. Remember, it
is not your fault. No-one should be subjected to this behaviour. It is okay to
walk away to protect your mental health.

The Workaholic They live and breathe their academic work and therefore are working all the time, and expect that of you too. They may (incorrectly) equate work hours with passion.

How to manage this behaviour: Setting boundaries is paramount (see Chap. 4). Be firm and provide dates of when you will deliver on work. It may be necessary to ignore not-so-subtle "comments" about your working hours.

The "Means well" One of the most difficult supervisory styles to deal with is actually a supervisor that "means well" but often misses the mark. Perhaps they struggle to give positive feedback, or are often so overburdened you come last on their "to-do list".

How to manage this behaviour: Given they likely care about your success, it is important to be upfront with your supervisor and explain to them that you need a different management style, or that things aren't quite working for you. This is mutually beneficial.

9.7 Pervasive, Damaging Biases

Unfortunately, some PhD Supervisors can carry some particularly damaging biases that can impact mental health heavily. They may see these entrenched biases as supportive when they are not.

Sink or Swim In order to "accelerate your learning" your supervisor may choose to give you little guidance and see how you cope. When you ask for help they may tell you to go away and think about the problem more. Whilst critical thinking is important for the PhD journey, if you knew exactly how to do everything before you started you would not need your supervisor in the first place. You will need assistance to succeed. The "Sink or Swim" mentality is toxic and is like putting someone out in the middle of the ocean on a boat but with no rowing equipment to get back to shore [17].

Suffering Is a Rite of Passage Another common toxic supervisory bias is taking the stance that "a PhD is meant to be hard" or "I suffered so you should too". This is unacceptable. A PhD is tough enough without unnecessary suffering on top of it. It can be difficult as a PhD student to understand the difference between being "pushed" and being abused due to the power dynamic, but you should never be made to feel uncomfortable or belittled in any way [18].

I Did It, so You Can too An example of survivorship or survival bias,[4] those that make it to professorial positions can fall back on the idea that if they have been successful then you can be too [19]. Whilst this could be perceived as positive, in many cases it results in the overlooking of obstacles that the PhD student may be experiencing that were not present when the PhD Supervisor did their PhD due to privilege or a change in the PhD landscape since they did their PhD.

Your Wellbeing Is Not My Problem A common notion is that pastoral care is not the responsibility of the supervisor [20]. This is not true, but it can make it difficult to receive any non-academic support from your supervisor. It can also mean that if you open up about your mental health you may not get the support you require.

Note: these beliefs, sadly are often not going to change. But I hope by being aware of them you may be able to recognise them if you are experiencing them and realise that you are not at fault.

9.8 When Things Go Seriously Wrong (and It Is Definitely Not Your Fault)

Unfortunately bullying and harassment is rife within academia. 43% of researchers stated they had experienced bullying and harassment, while 61% had witnessed it [21, 22]. Of those, 59% of those that had experienced it said the perpetrator was a supervisor. Below are some examples of supervisors bullying, harassing and/or manipulating their PhD students. This is absolutely not okay and if you are experiencing these things you are in a toxic situation. Some examples of abuses of power and inappropriate conduct include [23–25]:

- Overlooking contributions/passing off your ideas as their own.
- Being verbally abused in group meetings.
- Shouting or raising their voice at you.
- Exclusion from academic publications or denial of proper author list placement.
- Asking for favours, sexual or otherwise.
- Attempting to start a romantic relationship with you.

---

[4] Survivor bias is defined as the logical error of concentrating on the people or things that made it past some selection process and overlooking those that did not, typically because of their lack of visibility.

- Telling you to doctor or edit research to support their opinion.
- Contacting you regularly outside of work on your personal number.
- Using a VISA application/right to work as leverage over you.
- Threatening to deport you if you do not comply.
- Keeping your passport/identity documents for "safe keeping".
- Forcing you to work on National/Bank holidays.
- Making you work routinely more than the allotted hours in a day.
- Holding you back from graduating for cheap labour.
- Not allowing you time out of your schedule to attend medical appointments.

Now whilst some of these may seem extreme, I assure you they do happen. If you have been victim to any of these sorts of behaviours (or similar), I want to reiterate that this is **not your fault**. You deserve to be treated with dignity and respect. *Note: More information on reporting these behaviours and what support is available to you is available in the online resources accompanying the book.*

> My supervisor gave me a project that wasn't getting results. He threatened to fire me (and revoke my visa) if I didn't get the results he wanted in 3 months. He forbade me to speak about this to anyone because he said "things would go very wrong" for me.—PhD Student 41

9.9 What You Can Do If Your Supervisor Is Abusive

Dealing with scenarios where your supervisor is abusive can be incredibly difficult due to the power dynamic at work. In many cases abuse goes unreported for this reason. There are however possible routes for you to manage the situation you find yourself in [26]:

Confide in Someone Whether it is a colleague, postdoc, academic you respect at your institution or friends/family, reach out to someone (if you can) and let them know what has been happening. Again, I want to reiterate that how you have been treated is not your fault and you deserve to be helped.

Keep a Record If the abuse is pervasive and frequent, keep a log of any written records of the behaviour that you have, as well as note down any witnesses present in meetings where abuse occurred.

Speak to Your Graduate School Whether it is your committee chair (US) or second supervisor (EU) there are formal reporting routes for supervisor misconduct. Often you can have informal, off the record conversations to understand the options that you have available to you. *Note: It is important to realise in some cases speaking to someone higher up in the university may mean word of your conversation getting back to your supervisor.*

Change Supervisor If your mental health and wellbeing is being heavily impacted by your supervisor it may be time to consider changing supervisor. This can be an incredibly difficult decision, particularly if you are already part way through your PhD. You must consider whether or not you can tolerate working for your supervisor for the time you have left on your PhD. The sunk-cost fallacy[5] can lead us to think that we should not change. *Note: To start this process, you would typically have to have a conversation with your course coordinator or graduate school. External transfers are possible, depending on funding.*

Speak to Your Union For impartial advice, representation and understanding of your workers' rights, Unions are invaluable, as well as Graduate Student Associations. It is often not known that PhD students are able to join organisations like University and College Union (UCU).

Know It Is Okay to Walk Away You should not have to walk away in a fair world, but if your mental health is at risk, know it is more than okay to step away from the situation you find yourself in.

9.10 Effective Communication

A large portion of your relationship with your supervisor is going to be dictated by your ability to communicate with one another. Understanding what motivates your supervisor can make a massive difference. Many PhD Supervisors are under constant pressure to output publications and bring in funding grants, with this being a vicious cycle; the more papers the more grants, the more papers, the more grants, etc. Thus their focus is going to primarily be on output. It can often feel that in an ideal world, based on

---

[5] The sunk cost fallacy reasoning states that *further investments or commitments are justified because the resources already invested will be lost otherwise.* In the case of PhD study it can be that if we just "stick it out" and try to manage the abuse we are being subject to we will get our PhD. In reality, leaving and starting a PhD elsewhere may be beneficial.

output, a PhD Supervisor would want to have a student that "just gets on with things", requiring little input from them, but this is not how the PhD process works. If you already knew how to do a PhD there would be no point in having a PhD Supervisor in the first place, as you would be able to complete it without their input. At the end of the day you are a student, and are learning. You will need (and are entitled to) help from your supervisor and the additional training provided by your doctoral program to ensure you succeed.

Thankfully, most PhD Supervisors are well-intentioned and care about their PhD students. Even so, it is important for us to realise that they are humans too, and under pressure they may not do a perfect job. They are also likely managing a range of different students (and personalities) which can be a difficult task. Thus, in order to build a successful relationship, and get the support you need, you may have to "manage upwards" [27]. This is an essential skill—useful well beyond your doctorate—as whilst you cannot control how your supervisor may react to certain situations, through effective communication you may be able to influence their management style to better suit you. So how might you go about this?

Understand What You Need Before communicating with your supervisor, consider what it is that you actually need. This sounds simple, but you will only get a clear response if you ask a clear question. It is also okay to ask for general guidance on what your next steps should be as you are a student and you are learning [28].

Realise They Will Always Be Busy Putting your needs first can be difficult, particularly when you are in awe of your PhD Supervisor. You may feel you don't want to "trouble" them until their schedule slows down a bit, but in reality, it likely never will. By taking on a PhD student they have committed to supporting you, so organise that meeting.

Operate with the "Yes, but" Rule When given demands from your supervisor, such as "I need you to review this for me for Friday", using the "Yes, but" rule can be helpful. For example, "Yes, but this means that I will not be able to get my presentation done by Wednesday as I will need to take time for the review.", helps to set realistic boundaries.

Be Direct PhD Supervisors have designated time to speak to their PhD students, so make sure to be direct and ask for what you need in any correspondence upfront. This will of course depend on your relationship dynamics and the personality of your supervisor to a certain extent. *Tip: It is important to* *realise that direct and aggressive are different things. It is okay to be assertive. Make sure that you include "please" and "thank you" accordingly.*

Outline Expectations If you need your PhD Supervisor to review a document for you, or provide feedback by a certain date, do not be afraid to give them the dates and state directly what you need from them. Being organised will help your supervisor stay on track.

Do Not Be Afraid to Ask Twice It may be that your email gets read and accidently forgotten about, or pushed down the priority list of your PhD Supervisor, but getting their feedback might be the limiting step for you to progress. Sending a follow up email is often reasonable and may remind them to look at your work.

9.11 What to Do if You Have a Disagreement

When doing research, disagreements on research interpretations are not uncommon [29]. This can be difficult to manage if it is your PhD Supervisor you are disagreeing with. For the most part professional disagreements will likely resolve on their own, and may even build rapport with your PhD Supervisor, as debate is part of the learning process. Often there is also no "right" or "wrong" with research either, just different approaches.

However, sometimes disagreements can turn nasty and as we have discussed earlier in this chapter, the power imbalance between PhD student and PhD Supervisor can be tough to navigate. Possible resolutions include:

Remember Their Expertise It is important to remember that your PhD Supervisor has a lot of experience in their area of specialty. Make sure to listen to their point of view. It is also important to realise that they can be wrong— they are only human after all.

Collect Proof No-one is going to know more about the daily ins and outs of what you do than you. If your PhD Supervisor is unconvinced by your arguments, obtaining proof from literature or by running experiments to prove your theory may be necessary.

Determine if It Has Become Ad Hominem If the disagreement has started to move away from a professional discussion, and more towards a personal attack, this is a red flag. You may want to call out this behaviour (if you feel able to) or report this to someone within your department.

They Don't Like to Be Challenged Questioning research methods and direction, and proposing other solutions are all part of the PhD journey. If you are hitting a huge amount of resistance, consider asking for reasons why your PhD Supervisor's direction is the preferred one. If the answer is along the lines of "just do it" or "I am calling the shots", this may be a sign your PhD Supervisor is not supportive. You should be able to ask questions.

> I disagreed with the direction of my PhD and voiced my concerns to my PhD Supervisor. They told me to just get on with the work and "quit whining". I ended up wasting 6 months of my PhD on something that was never going to work because they wouldn't listen.—PhD Student 42

In rare cases disagreements can result in the relationship between a PhD Student and PhD Supervisor to break down irrevocably. If you think you have reached this point during your PhD, I strongly recommend considering moving PhD group or changing PhD Supervisor. If they do not have your best interests at heart it is going to be an uphill struggle to get your PhD. In some uncommon situations, PhD Supervisors may have an active vendetta against a student as they challenged them. This is unacceptable behaviour. *Note: The online resource that accompanies this book has information on how to report this behaviour if you feel able.*

ADVOCATING FOR BETTER: What Can Universities Do to Improve PhD Supervision?

Given the professional relationship between PhD Supervisor and PhD student can have such broad implications for research output and PhD completion, in my opinion, institutions must make sure to:

1. **Monitor and look at drop-out rate:** Is there a supervisor who's students are dropping out at greater rates than average? This should be explored to understand if there is a problem with the supervisor and the research culture that they foster.
2. **Provide training:** Being good at research does not necessarily mean being good at being a mentor. Specific training and outlining of expectations for PhD Supervisors must be provided. Refresher courses are also essential as what is required of a supervisor and ways of managing change over time.
3. **Make sure support is signposted:** Typically useful university mental health support exists, but this does not mean that supervisors know where resources are, how to access them, and direct students towards them. Support must be clear and accessible.

(continued)

(continued)

4. **Provide mental health support for supervisors:** If a supervisor is struggling with their own mental health it can be tough to provide support for others. Making sure that they know the range of support available and where to access it is important.
5. **Student-supervisor agreement [30]:** A student-supervisor agreement established at the start of a PhD program can help to outline expectations for both parties and be used to hold individuals accountable if they do not live up to their end of the bargain. For example, explicitly stating working hours so that students feel that they can say no if asked to work extreme hours.
6. **Consider exit interviews:** Anonymised exit interviews can provide a way to get feedback from students and understand the working conditions that they have been exposed to. *Note: Care needs to be taken to ensure that retaliation cannot happen, for example only discussing data after several years to avoid identification.*

Perhaps most important, is to recognise that from an institutional perspective, in the short term it may seem like protecting a PhD Supervisor that brings in a lot of funding is financially more lucrative, than to hold them accountable, but long term the damage that can be done by one individual is huge, from driving out talented individuals from academia, to wide-scale institutional reputation damage. The former in my opinion is much more important.

References

1. van Rooij E, Fokkens-Bruinsma M, Jansen E (2021) Factors that influence PhD candidates' success: the importance of PhD project characteristics. Stud Contin Educ 43(1):48–67
2. Woolston C (2019) PhDs: the tortuous truth. Nature 575(7782):403–407
3. Pyke KD (2018) Institutional betrayal: inequity, discrimination, bullying, and retaliation in academia. Sociol Perspect 61(1):5–13
4. Vilkinas T (1998) Management of the PhD process: the challenging role of the supervisor. In: Quality in postgraduate research. University of Adelaide, Adelaide
5. Rose GL (2003) Enhancement of mentor selection using the ideal mentor scale. Res High Educ 44(4):473–494
6. Vilkinas T, Cartan G (2006) The integrated competing values framework: its spatial configuration. J Manage Dev 25(6):505–521
7. Guccione K, Hutchinson S (2021) Coaching and mentoring for academic development. Emerald Group, Bingley
8. Hund AK, Churchill AC, Faist AM, Havrilla CA, Stowell SML, McCreery HF, Ng J, Pinzone CA, Scordato ESC (2018) Transforming mentorship in STEM by training scientists to be better leaders. Ecol Evol 8(20):9962–9974

9. Amundsen C, McAlpine L (2009) 'Learning supervision': trial by fire. Innov Educ Teach Int 46(3):331–342

10. Schimanski LA, Alperin JP (2018) The evaluation of scholarship in academic promotion and tenure processes: past, present, and future. F1000Research 71605

11. Bagilhole B (1993) How to keep a good woman down: an investigation of the role of institutional factors in the process of discrimination against women academics. Br J Sociol Educ 14(3):261–274

12. Aiston SJ, Jung J (2015) Women academics and research productivity: an international comparison. Gend Educ 27(3):205–220

13. Giacalone RA, Knouse SB, Montagliani A (1997) Motivation for and prevention of honest responding in exit interviews and surveys. J Psychol 131(4):438–448

14. Hall W, Liva S (2022) Falling through the cracks: graduate students' experiences of mentoring absence. Can J Scholarsh Teach Learn 13(1):1–15

15. UK Research Councils Statement of Expectations for Postgraduate Training. https://www.ukri.org/wp-content/uploads/2021/07/UKRI-120721-StatementOfExpectationsPostGradTraining.pdf. Accessed 21 Jun 2022

16. Chamberlain S (2016) Ten types of PhD supervisor relationships - which is yours? https://theconversation.com/ten-types-of-phd-supervisor-relationships-which-is-yours-52967. Accessed 21 Jun 2022

17. Clay M (2012) Sink or swim: drowning the next generation of research leaders? Aust Q 83(4):26–31

18. Bégin C, Géarard L (2013) The role of supervisors in light of the experience of doctoral students. Policy Futures Educ 11(3):267–276

19. Hemprich-Bennett D, Rabaiotti D, Kennedy E (2021) Beware survivorship bias in advice on science careers. Nature 598(7880):373–374

20. Parker-Jenkins M (2018) Mind the gap: developing the roles, expectations and boundaries in the doctoral supervisor–supervisee relationship. Stud High Educ 43(1):57–71

21. Moran H, Karlin L, Lauchlan E, Rappaport SJ, Bleasdale B, Wild L, Dorr J (2020) Understanding research culture: what researchers think about the culture they work in. Wellcome Trust, London, UK

22. Lee D (1998) Sexual harassment in PhD supervision. Gend Educ 10(3):299–312

23. Misawa M (2015) Cuts and bruises caused by arrows, sticks, and stones in academia: theorizing three types of racist and homophobic bullying in adult and higher education. Adult Learn 26(1):6–13

24. Cohen A, Baruch Y (2021) Abuse and exploitation of doctoral students: a conceptual model for traversing a long and winding road to academia. J Bus Ethics:1–18

25. Moss SE, Mahmoudi M (2021) STEM the bullying: an empirical investigation of abusive supervision in academic science. EClinicalMedicine 40101121

26. Gewin V (2021) How to blow the whistle on an academic bully. Nature 593(7858):299–301

27. Saló-Salgado L, Acocella A, Arzuaga García I, El Mousadik S, and Zvinavashe A (2021) Managing up: how to communicate effectively with your PhD adviser. https://www.nature.com/articles/d41586-021-03703-z. Accessed 15 Feb 2022

28. The Wellbeing Thesis (2022) Managing your supervisor. https://thewellbeingthesis.org.uk/using-the-resources-available/managing-your-supervisor/. Accessed 20 Feb 2022

29. Eley A, Jennings R (2005) Effective postgraduate supervision: improving the student/supervisor relationship. McGraw-Hill Education (UK), London, UK

30. Hockey J (1996) A contractual solution to problems in the supervision of PhD degrees in the UK. Stud High Educ 21(3):359–371

10

Publish or Perish: On the Myth of Meritocracy

The fact that "Publish or Perish" exists as a term at all in academia tells us a lot about academic culture. In the pursuit of academic "excellence", the fact we are human can often get lost along the way. Instead, from day one, focus is placed on output—be it publications, collaborations, or conducting experiments. The larger and more innovative the output, the more "successful" we are deemed to be. Papers are perhaps best likened to being universal currency in academia; the more papers you get the more you are likely to get an academic position going forward. It follows that a large amount of pressure arises around trying to get as many high-impact publications as possible during your PhD journey. This is further compounded by the fact that publications are often placed on a higher pedestal than other work within the academy, such as mentoring, outreach, collegiate work, diversity and inclusion initiatives, and teaching, despite these other aspects of academic positions having huge impact on the retention of future researchers. This is a clear systemic issue.

Not all academic research is considered equal either, with evaluation criteria such as "Research Excellence Framework" (REF) in the UK being used by institutions to determine the impact of outputted research. This system has been criticised for considering "groundbreaking" research as higher quality than studies looking at replicating findings or exploring incremental changes, despite replication of results being a huge cornerstone of the scientific method [1]. This adds huge pressure onto researchers to constantly innovate, and find novel research avenues to explore.

(Trigger Warnings: bullying)

© The Author(s), under exclusive license to Springer Nature Switzerland AG 2022
Z. J. Ayres, *Managing your Mental Health during your PhD*,
https://doi.org/10.1007/978-3-031-14194-2_10

It follows then that in the back of your mind, there will likely always be a niggling feeling of "I should be doing more", because theoretically, the more time you put in, the more likely you are to generate publishable work and new ideas. This underpins the pervasive culture of overwork in academia. Feeling the need to constantly be "on" all the time can lead to lack of sleep, increased stress, feelings of inadequacy, and anxiety over whether you will publish any outputs during your PhD program, all impacting mental health. In reality, there is of course a limit to how much of our time and energy that we can put into chasing publications—if we give too much we will reach burnout which can impact our creativity and prevent us from doing work entirely. This itself is a vicious circle as that can then impede getting publications. A balance is therefore needed, which can be tough to find.[1] It is also clear that maintaining good mental health in this scenario can be difficult.

What we can end up doing is constantly worrying about our future and the person we would have been "if I had just worked last weekend rather than doing X", where X might be relaxing, spending time with our family, or simply resting. I likely cannot help you through these feelings of guilt in their entirety, but I do want to remind you that you not only deserve rest, you are entitled to it. Further, we have to let go of the "What if?" version of us—that "perfect" version of us that pushed on through and did research every hour of every waking day. They simply are not real. It's only when we realise this that we can start to work with ourselves and look at the tools we have at our disposal (like self-care) and find the balance between research output and looking after our wellbeing that we need to thrive.

In this chapter, what I cannot do is fix the current heavy weighting on publications within the university system. It is clearly a systemic issue that fuels overwork, hyper-competition and poor work-life balance. One of the tools I can give you though is a deeper understanding of how the publication process works and help you feel a little bit more comfortable with the process, helping to alleviate some concerns you may have.

---

[1] I know I found this particularly difficult, as I constantly worried that if I didn't "keep up" then future me would be somehow hamstringed when trying to get future positions. I now realise that focusing on future me without giving any care for current me is not sustainable.

10.1   It Is Not an Equal Playing Field

One of the biggest misconceptions that we tend to have as PhD students when starting our PhD program is that by putting in hard work and as many hours as physically possible, we will generate academic publications. In reality there are many other contributors going on behind the scenes:

Luck A huge factor in whether or not we get publishable results throughout our PhD is luck. The particular research area we explore may not have an outcome that is publishable, and this is outside of our control. This is always the case with frontier research, as we are exploring and unknown space. Unfortunately (in STEM subjects) this leads to the possibility of our findings being null. *Note: it is important to remember that a null result is still a result, it might just not be the game-changing find we were hoping for. The contribution of luck often goes unmentioned because those that have/are successful would love everyone to believe that they achieved based on grit alone (spoiler: they absolutely did not).*

Privilege If we think back to getting papers being like currency, some individuals may have an advantage. For example, they may have had a family member already get a doctorate, which can help understand what is required when it comes to publications. Further, not everyone can work late into evenings, or all weekend, because they have other jobs to do, caring responsibilities, or need to manage their mental health, thus take time away from academia. Those that do not have these, gain an advantage [2]. Coming from a richer socioeconomic group can also be the difference between having a weekly cleaner, or buying in healthy ready meals enabling more time to do research.[2] This is a complex problem, as if certain marginalised groups can never reach the same output as other colleagues (due to caring responsibilities for example), but bring a different, valuable perspective, the whole "success" criteria that academia models is not actually favourable towards diverse talent retention.

Access to Equipment/Data A sub-set of privilege, not every university has the same access to equipment as others. This may particularly affect STEM PhD students. It may mean that there is a long wait on using equipment that

---

[2] I remember a scientific talk I went to where the professor presenting was asked how they did it all, as they had an established research career as well as six children. Not once did they mention their wife working as a full-time mother, despite this being the case, enabling them to do their research.

you need, or that you may have to travel to a different university entirely to do some of your studies. This is likely to slow your progress, and is outside your control. Access to data may also be easier at some institutions than others, due to wealthier universities paying for more data processing software, or even being more well-known to the general population so that they are more likely to come forward as participants for studies. Universities based in Low and Middle Income Countries (LMIC) may be particularly impacted.

Field The area in which you are studying in (and even sub-set of your field) may dictate the number of publications you are likely to achieve during your PhD. For example if you require ethical approval this may slow down the process. Further, the impact factor of journals you publish in is also topic dependent. Depending on your area of study, publishing papers may not be considered as important as publishing a book, monograph or producing other outputs.

Who You Know For the most part the peer review process is not anonymised. This means that the editors and reviewers will know what research group submitted the paper for review, as well as the names of the authors. This opens up the paper publishing process to bias. This could be bias against the gender of the paper authors, against the country of origin, or the PI on the paper etc. For example, the Institute of Physics found that papers with female corresponding authors were found to have a lower acceptance rate than those from male corresponding authors (40% compared to 43% acceptance rate respectively) [3]. Whilst this may seem like a small difference, it still carries a knock-on effect.

So now you know all this, it is clear that not everyone starts on the same playing field. Not everyone has the same access and privilege as everyone else. Nor do they have equal chance of success when it comes to academic publications. Many of us are brought up to believe that if we "just try hard enough" we can succeed. This isn't the case. *Academia is not a meritocracy.*

Publishing Costs Depending on the journal publishing costs can be huge sums of money (even/especially publishing research open access, which is somewhat ironic). These costs mean that for some institutions, publishing in some journals is not possible. For research groups with smaller pots of available funds this may also limit the number of publications that get published each year. *Note: You should never be asked to cover the publishing costs of a paper* *yourself, as an individual. These costs should always be covered by your institution. Further, predatory publishers may write to you and ask you to contribute your work to their journal for a fee—this is generally a scam and should be ignored. Legitimate requests for contributions to special editions of journals are likely to be directed at your PhD Supervisor.*

This all can seem deflating at first, but it is important to realise that it is largely *outside your control*. Once you accept that fact you can move on to focus on what you *can control*, to help you throughout the PhD process, and beat the odds. For what it is worth, your publication record, whilst important, is not a measure of your ability. As I stated at the start of this book though, I do want you to succeed in academia. And if we have to operate within the "norms" of academia and the current definition of what success looks like, It is important to effectively manage our mental health so that we can have the energy to pursue research, and get as much research output as possible.

10.2   The Publication Process

If there's one bit of advice I can give you on the pressure to publish it is that publishable work comes with time. You may not get data to be able to publish anything in the first year or two of your PhD, and as we get further into our PhD and understand the field, output tends to increase over time. Even then, depending on how challenging your project is, creating a tangible narrative out of only small parts of a bigger jigsaw puzzle can be tough, if not impossible. This does not mean that your work has no value, just that you are contributing to a larger picture that may require decades more work to truly understand. This is the nature of research.

Understanding how the publication process works can go some of the way to helping alleviate some of the worries and anxieties you might feel about the process. Whilst these will be slightly different journal to journal, the general outline of the publication process is illustrated in Fig. 10.1.

Once your paper is submitted there are a range of possible options as to what happens next. The first is a "desk reject" from the editor of the journal that you submitted your manuscript to. This is where the paper does not go out to reviewers in your field as the editor believes that the manuscript that has been submitted is not within scope of the journal. When this happens, it may be due to a calculated risk (aiming for a high-impact journal with the hope it may be accepted, despite knowing there is a high chance that it may get rejected), or not quite pitching the research to the right journal. These are

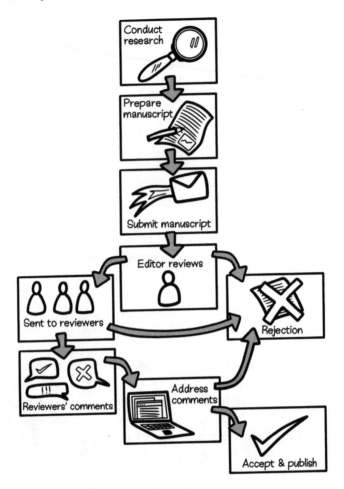

Fig. 10.1 Flow diagram of the typical publication process

both things that an experienced PhD Supervisor should prepare you for. If a desk reject does happen to you, not all hope is lost. Although disheartening, and often involving a few extra days/weeks of work, most manuscripts can be edited and re-prepared to submit elsewhere. It is also worth noting that some journals may only want to publish articles that are very different to other articles that they have published. Thus, if there is some similarities between your work and another paper, the journal may make a decision not to publish based on novelty, even if they are different pieces of work. This does not mean your work is not publishable, just that another journal might be more appropriate.

When a paper is approved by a journal editor, the next stage is the paper being sent out for review to other experts in the field. You may be asked to supply reviewer recommendations, although this does not guarantee that your paper will be sent to the people you have chosen (if this was always the case there is the possibility of bias, with friends in the field reviewing and approving other friends papers, if conducted unethically). The review process can take several months (or longer), and the uncertainty at this stage can be tough to manage. *Tip: Whilst your paper is out for review it is no longer in your control. To this end, if possible, try to use your energy on other research rather than worrying about the outcome.*

After the reviewers' have had a chance to review your manuscript, the editor will then pass these comments back to you. At this stage there are several outcomes: publish without revision, publish with revision, and reject.

Receiving a rejection sucks. I don't think there is a better or more polite way to say it. It is also highly likely to happen at some point during your PhD research. It's okay to take a moment to feel and collect your thoughts when rejection happens—it is not a nice feeling, particularly when it is on something you have worked hard on for several years. On receiving a rejection— the real work begins by asking "Why has this happened?" and working with your PhD Supervisor to make changes to your manuscript. The most important thing to remember is that (for the most part) rejections are not personal, and are simply trying to ensure novelty within your research field.

Publishing with revision, involves getting feedback on the manuscript from the reviewers with key items to address in order to ensure that the paper is fit for publication. Once all comments are addressed, typically, on returning to the editor, the paper will then be accepted (or rejected in a small number of cases). *Note: The "Resources" section of this book links out to a range of guides on how to write and edit papers for publication.*

10.3 Managing Reviewer 2

Constructive comments serve to improve the manuscript and the result is often a better, more detailed piece of work after addressing reviewers comments. However, you may have heard of the notorious "Reviewer 2" [4]. This is used as a euphemism for receiving critical comments on a manuscript from a reviewer. Whilst reviewers should always be respectful and polite, unfortunately this is not always the case. It is necessary to consider whether or not the comments made are constructive. It is easy to forget that reviewers also carry biases (and grudges) and unfortunately (in rare cases) reviewing manuscripts can be misused to hurt others. Whilst some journals are now working towards anonymised peer review process, many have yet to take this approach. If feedback is cruel it is important to remember that it really is the reviewers problem, not yours. It may be possible in this instance to appeal any decisions on a manuscript to the journal editor. Ultimately, whilst this can be a setback, and should not happen, it is highly likely you will find another journal to publish your work in. Further, it is possible to contend the reviewers comments. For example, rerunning an experiment might take another 6 months, and might not be feasible. Thus there is some flexibility on what comments are addressed or not. *Tip: Being a reviewer yourself may give you valuable insight to the reviewing process and give you an opportunity to improve a range of skills for your CV. You are often automatically signed up to be part of a reviewer pool after your first publication.*

10.4   Publishing Options

As you near the end of your PhD the pressure to publish can really begin to mount. Publishing may not be an option, or it may seem that there simply is not enough time left. Some options include:

Seek Collaborations Doing a full research project on your own is a big and daunting task. If possible, teaming up with others that have different skillsets/ perspectives to help complete bodies of work, can lead to faster output and more rigorous research.

Consider Pre-prints If you are nearing the end of your PhD, pre-print servers may be a good option to get your research out into the public domain before formal publication. This also negates papers getting held up in months of review, without the wider research community having access to the work. Further, this provides opportunity to not only get feedback from the reviewers on your manuscript, but also other independent researchers. This can be invaluable for making changes and strengthening the final publication. *Note: some funding bodies/journals may not approve of pre-prints so this needs to be checked first.*

Know It Is Okay to Finish Up Publications After Graduating As much as we would like to have everything neatly wrapped up and in publications when we finish our PhD programs, the chances are you will not achieve this. In a sense, this is a good thing because it means that there is much more research stemming from the work you have done. It is important to remember that you will be able to work on and submit papers after you finish your PhD, and if you do not have time afterwards, manuscripts will be finished by others.

I didn't publish during my PhD and I'm now 7 months into my postdoc (still having not published anything!) it takes time and shouldn't be rushed!—Postdoctoral Researcher 1

10.5   Who Is Perishing, Anyway?

As we will discuss in more detail in the next chapter, the majority of PhD students do not go on to stay in university roles, they instead go on to work in industry, government roles, and non-profit organisations, to name just a few. "Perish" quite literally means to "suffer complete ruin or destruction", which is quite frankly overly dramatic and not true. It is easy to think about an alternate timeline version of ourselves that worked through the night and managed to get 12 first author publications in top journals, but that is not sustainable for anyone other than a robot. For many of us with mental illness, putting our wellbeing first is not so much a choice, but our only option to stay well.

I had no first author papers leaving my PhD and [am] now about to start my own lab.—Early Career Academic 1

It is important to remember, without you there would be no PhD. Whilst publications are often considered currency in academia, they are not the be all and end all. Further, some jobs post-PhD may not care about the number of publications you have at all.

I was on several papers during my PhD, 4 of which were first author. When I interviewed for industrial positions after I decided to leave academia they really did not care about the number or quality of my publications. The focus was on my skillset.—Industry Scientist 1

It is clear that cultural change within academia is also needed to recognise skills that contribute to academia outside the publication of papers. This is happening slowly. There needs to be more recognition for pastoral care, mentorship, compassion, and many more "soft skills"[3] that make great researchers.

10.6   Perfectionism

Perfectionism can also trickle in during the publication process, making it difficult to actually submit a manuscript. This can largely stem from fear of rejection. It is important to remember that any piece of research work is an evolving story, and that it will never be "complete". This is where "good enough" comes in. Further, reviewers are always going to look for "holes" in your manuscript—this is their job—so it is highly unlikely you will submit the perfect manuscript. One could even argue that if you did submit the perfect manuscript and got glowing reviewers comments, perhaps that was time that could have been spent on other research has been spent finalising the manuscript (something if you are working towards a time sensitive PhD should be avoided). *Tip: A written draft is better than nothing written on a page. Start with bullet points to outline your main messages and build from there. Also useful is to keep all draft writing (even bits you delete) saved in a document so you can go back and use sentences you wrote at a later date.*

10.7   Writing Your Thesis

Of course, the biggest publication output you will have during your PhD is your thesis (or dissertation). This is one of the most challenging times during a PhD due to a range of factors, from feeling like condensing all the work you did over the last few years is an insurmountable task, to struggling with motivation, to feeling isolated. There are a range of fantastic guides out there for how to write a PhD thesis that do a much better job exploring strategies to get you through the write-up portion of your PhD than I can here (please see the online resources recommended online, accompanying this book [5]), but here are a few thoughts on how you might manage some of the feelings you may be experiencing during the write-up phase:

---

[3] I personally do not see these as "soft skills" at all, but essential skills needed for true people leaders.

Feeling Overwhelmed If possible start planning your thesis and work on chunks early (but please do not panic if you have not done this). Discuss a thesis outline with your PhD Supervisor, and look at what work is outstanding, making a priority list. Break down the work into manageable chunks, or set yourself a writing target of so many words per day. If you are running research studies/experiments still, decide where your stopping point is.[4]

Feeling Isolated It can be really tempting to withdraw from socialising when writing up, and spending time in your own writing bubble. If possible, try to avoid doing this completely. You may benefit from working in a coffee shop or library for some human interaction.

Feeling Unmotivated It is completely natural to feel unmotivated at times. It may seem counterintuitive, but consider stepping away for a bit and having a break if you can. Switching up what you are working on can also help. For example, working on a figure, or formatting, rather than writing for a while. Online writing communities to assist with accountability may help.

Feeling Panicked A hard, looming deadline can be a scary thing, especially when your PhD is at stake. It is important to remember that you are the expert in your field, and that there is a range of support available to you, from colleagues to the online community. Extensions may be possible if needed.

Feeling Indifferent One of the most difficult feelings to manage is not feeling or caring much about your PhD. I have both experienced this and seen others go through this. Try to look at this logically: that finish line is not far away, and the power is yours to get there.

If all else fails, remember, you've got this, you are the expert in this work. You *can* do this.

10.8 Research Misconduct

The Committee for Publication Ethics (COPE) states that "good research should be well adjusted, well-planned, appropriately designed, and ethically approved. To conduct research to a lower standard may constitute misconduct

---

[4] I found knowing where to stop running experiments very difficult as there is always more work to be done, and more detailed conclusions to be made with more data. But at some point you have to draw the line.

[6, 7]." Yet, the pressure to publish in academia can have dire consequences, as in academia papers are like currency, with the focus on output, quantity over quality an increasing problem. And for some, this leads to research misconduct. This has also led to the "replication crisis" in STEM. This is where data within (predominantly scientific) publications, is not repeatable, even if a person trying to replicate the data follows all the instructions outlined in the methods section to the letter. In some cases, this is because the authors are in such a rush to publish that they abandon all rigour and do not replicate their work. But unfortunately there is also a more sinister underlying problem throughout research: data manipulation. In some cases, the pressure to publish results in individuals abandoning their integrity and manipulating data to suit their hypothesis. This is research misconduct, is unethical, and can result in reputations being ruined if discovered. Over the last few years, the award winning microbiologist and data manipulation sleuth Dr Elisabeth Bik has found thousands of cases of suspected results tampering and instigated over 150 paper retractions, and it is thought that there are many yet to be discovered [8].[5] Unfortunately data manipulation is not just the act of individuals either. There is evidence that some PhD Supervisors may embed academic misconduct within their research groups, pass it off as normal and make it difficult for students to refuse due to the inherent power dynamic that exists. This can have huge implications for mental health.

There is no excuse for this behaviour, but it can be really challenging to navigate as a PhD student. Ethical violations look like [9]:

- Not declaring conflicts of interest.
- Plagiarism (including self-plagiarism).
- Omitting authors that contributed to work off research papers.
- Adding authors that did not contribute to research papers.
- Not obtaining ethical approval for studies.
- Manipulating/altering data.
- Asking leading questions.
- Publishing redundant work (publishing the same paper with title changed).
- Collecting data on human participants without respect and dignity.
- Poor handling of sensitive information/anonymity.
- Rerunning of data until the result that is "wanted" is obtained.

---

[5] Work by Bik is based largely on image forensics, detecting when an image has been manipulated, so this means that there is likely a whole host of other data manipulation out there where edits have been made to raw data sets that may never be uncovered.

10.9 What to Do if You Realise Research Misconduct Is Happening

If you find yourself in a situation where you feel pressured by someone to do something unethical, remember that you are the most likely person to suffer the consequences if you do it.

> My PhD Supervisor tried to force me to falsify data to support her hypothesis several times. She also tried to make me use a method that produced false results, and would not let me present anything during one-on-one meetings, or group meetings using the accurate method until I wasted a year of my PhD to show her that she was wrong. She begrudgingly admitted it. Every meeting she would tear into me to the point where I was having anxiety attacks before meetings, and in my personal life.—PhD Student 43

This doesn't mean all hope is lost if you have altered data at the request of someone in power because you felt you had no choice or didn't realise the ethical ramifications ahead of time. If you feel like you are trapped, know that it is never too late to be honest. Whistleblowing may lead to complete breakdown in the relationship between you and your PhD Supervisor, however your integrity as a researcher is far more important.

Here is a range of possible options available to you [10]:

Speak to Someone To start with this can be a heavy weight to carry, so consider confiding in a colleague about the situation. It may be that this has happened to other people in your research group too. Further, if you are worried about retaliation, speaking to someone outside of work like friends or family may be a good place to start.

Suggest Corrections [11] In some cases there might have been an error made through incompetence rather than intention. It may be a viable option to raise the issue and retract the work if needed.

Gather Evidence In order to create a formal complaint, documenting evidence of being asked to manipulate data is useful. This can include emails, as well as any conversation details you remember (including noting down if any witnesses were present). If you are being asked to manipulate data, explicitly asking the person to write that request down in an email is an option, for example: "Just to confirm, based on our conversation the other day you asked me to do X".

Join a Union/Speak to Your Graduate Office Most universities have a union or graduate office you can go to, although it is not always obvious that as a PhD student you are eligible to join staff unions. Unions act to protect the rights of workers and will be able to provide advice on what to do next, and may also be able to advocate for you.

Speak to Your Course Leader If you feel comfortable doing so, speak to your course leader about what has been happening. Make sure to keep a paper trail of correspondence. Unfortunately this is not without risk, as in some cases the institution may be protected not the student.

Find an Ally There may be another member of faculty in your department that you trust. Finding them and discussing your options with them before moving forward to more formal proceedings may help you get started.

Leaving the Program Honesty and integrity are two key parts of doing research. If the situation you find yourself in is untenable, the best option may be to walk away from the research group you are part of. This can be an incredibly difficult decision, but it is important to know that you will be incredibly competitive when applying for new PhD positions due to the experience you already have. You could also consider explaining the situation and why you left at interview.

ADVOCATING FOR BETTER: How Can the Pressure to Publish Be Improved for PhD Students?

With publication metrics so heavily attributed to success in academia, this can add huge pressure to PhD students. To provide support for this, in my opinion, institutions should:

1. **Encourage collaborations**—A collaborative working environment means that publishing papers does not require a PhD student to be an expert in all areas in order to publish their research. This (in theory) reduces the time it takes to publish work.
2. **Ensure that contributions are recognised**—Unfortunately there are many accounts of PhD students contributing to data collection/writing of publications and not getting credit on the paper for the work they did, due to biases and/or bullying. Clear, transparent procedures as to what contributes authorship should be in place.
3. **Demystify the publication process**—Do not assume that all PhD students understand the publication process, or will have it explained in detail to them by their supervisor. A lot of knowledge is assumed, but may not be there for first generation academics. Consider running training workshops for PhD students.
4. **Provide reporting routes for research misconduct**—Whilst we would all like to assume that scientific misconduct is not happening at our institutions, it likely is. Educating PhD students on what constitutes scientific misconduct as well as providing ways to report it is vital.
5. **Begin to recognise contributions outside of publications**—Systemic change in terms of what contributes "success" in academia needs to happen. It could be argued that there is a role to play from universities to ensure that output that is considered "successful" does not only include publications, but also inclusion and diversity work, teaching, pastoral responsibilities and more.

References

1. Jones A, Kemp A (2016) Why is so much research dodgy? Blame the Research Excellence Framework. The Guardian
2. Cech EA (2022) The intersectional privilege of white able-bodied heterosexual men in STEM. Sci Adv 8(24):eabo1558
3. Institute of Physics (2018) Diversity and inclusion in peer review at IOP publishing. IOP, London, UK
4. Watling C, Ginsburg S, Lingard L (2021) Don't be reviewer 2! Reflections on writing effective peer review comments. Perspect Med Educ 10(5):299–303
5. Dunleavy P (2003) Authoring a PhD: how to plan, draft, write and finish a doctoral thesis or dissertation. Bloomsbury, London
6. Jenn NC (2006) Common ethical issues in research and publication. Malays Fam Phys 1(2-3):74–76

7. Wager E (2012) The Committee on Publication Ethics (COPE): objectives and achievements 1997–2012. La Presse Medicale 41(9):861–866
8. Shen H (2020) Meet this super-spotter of duplicated images in science papers. Nature 581(7807):132–136
9. Marcovitch H (2007) Misconduct by researchers and authors. Gac Sanit 21(6):492–499
10. Wager E (2011) Coping with scientific misconduct. BMJ 343:d6586
11. Vie KJ (2020) How should researchers cope with the ethical demands of discovering research misconduct? Going beyond reporting and whistleblowing. Life Sci Soc Policy 16(6)

11

The High-Walled Rose Garden: Understanding There Is Life Outside the Academy

Understanding the job market and opportunities available post-PhD is essential to help navigate uncertainty around what comes next, as well as setting realistic expectations. Many of us go into doing a PhD with the expectation of becoming a professor one day, despite the fact that looking at the data, the probability is slim (Fig. 11.1).[1]

The data shows that in the United Kingdom, according to HESA Higher Education Student Statistics, the average number of enrolments in doctoral research was just over 100,000 students per year, from 2015 to 2020 [3]. Over the same time period the number of individuals employed at UK universities only increased by 1795 professorial positions from 2015 to 2020, with an average of ~16,600 positions in total [2]. This shows a huge disparity between the number of professorial positions and the cumulative PhD registrations each year. Further, given that the "change-over" of academics is slow (once someone has a professorship they are likely to stay in post for a decade or more, with over half of all professors aged 55 or over), the likelihood of becoming a professor drops even lower [4]. Of course not all jobs in academia are at professorial level, but even other teaching and research jobs that are available are significantly lower (~64,000), with a slow turnover rate, compared to PhD positions [2].

I do not tell you this to dishearten you, or to put you off pursuing your PhD. There are many reasons why we might do a PhD, including for the love of research, the academic freedoms it offers, as well as in some cases simply getting a fancy title we can use. I tell you to highlight to you that whilst a PhD

---

[1] Whilst this data is a little dated now, the likelihood is that this has only worsened further with time.

© The Author(s), under exclusive license to Springer Nature Switzerland AG 2022
Z. J. Ayres, *Managing your Mental Health during your PhD*,
https://doi.org/10.1007/978-3-031-14194-2_11

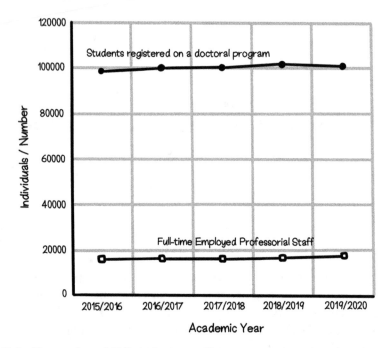

Fig. 11.1 The number of PhD students enrolling per year plotted against the number of professorial positions at UK universities, from 2015 to 2020, created from HESA data CC BY 4.0 [1, 2]

may seem like a good option for you, it does not guarantee a professorial position. However, knowing that the majority of PhD students do not become tenure-track professors, it is clear that they must end up working somewhere else[2]—i.e. you have options. By knowing how competitive the academic job market is, it is possible to build skills and ensure you have employability options that extend well beyond the academy.

This also means that expectations as to what makes a "good" academic has also changed, due to the high competition for positions. With the push to distinguish oneself from others in order to eventually join tenure track (or get a professorship in the UK), overwork has reared its ugly head and become normalised. Hyper-competition is perhaps the biggest driver of a toxic working culture within academia. It encourages overwork, with approximately 50% of PhD students reportedly working 51 hours or more per week, and 5%

---

[2] I would also be remiss not to mention that I myself transitioned from academia to industry after my first postdoctoral position came to an end. I found that the culture of overwork was unsustainable for me and maintaining good mental health. This is in part what has inspired me to continue to advocate for betting working conditions and improving the research culture in academia. I think it is important to acknowledge this because I carry my own biases along with this.

working greater than 80 hours [5]. This in and of itself is a health risk with EU working directive 2003/88/EC suggesting a maximum working week of 48 hours, because over this can be dangerous for both physical and mental health [6].

Further, data by the Royal Society suggests that only 0.45% of people that study in the sciences go on to become professors [7]. Whilst these data are primarily from Science, Technology, Engineering and Mathematics (STEM), a similar trend is seen within humanities, as observed through the Humanities Indicators Project, part of the American Academy of Arts and Sciences, which found that less than 30% of employed PhDs work in postsecondary education, with the rest leaving academia, with many joining legal, management, and business-orientated careers [8].

When looking at these statistics we must also consider the "success" rate of marginalised groups. This attrition rate is even worse for women in academia, with women only making up 28% of professorial staff in the UK (the so-called "leaky pipeline") [2]. Further, only 0.7% of UK university professors are Black [2]. This means that beating the odds and becoming a Professor is slim. This is changing though (albeit slowly), with increasing numbers of underrepresented groups advancing in academic spaces every year.

Concerningly, according to the Nature 2019 PhD Mental Health survey, whilst just over half of respondents felt that department staff were open to them pursuing a career outside of academia, only 29% said they had been given useful advice on this, and three quarters of respondents thought their program was not preparing them well for a non-research-related career [5]. This is why I think career uncertainty and understanding future career options are intrinsically related to PhD mental health, and are important to discuss in this book.

11.1 So What Does This Mean for You and Surviving Your PhD?

Those Giving You Advice May Not Know Any Different Repeatedly I see leaving academia described as "selling out" or that it is "a waste of a good mind" if someone goes to work somewhere else. But when we reflect on the individuals that say these statements, most of the time they have little to no experience of working outside of academia and thus they are making judgements based on knowing very little about the opportunities beyond the academy. This is the "high-walled rose garden". This means that those that have "made it" in academia, can only see the appeal of academia because they are actively inside it, and assume that life outside is worse. In some cases this is a self-preservation tactic; if you have dedicated your whole life to academia perhaps you do not want to know that your quality of life may have been equally good, or better outside of it.

You Can Succeed in Academia, but It May Come at a Cost To be "competitive" in a hypercompetitive environment is incredibly difficult. Overwork and managing mental illness is often not conducive to one another. This does not mean that success in academia is not possible, just that investment in mental health management and finding a supportive environment is essential.

In All Likelihood You Will Leave the Academy The statistics clearly show that at some time point you will likely leave the academy. Preparing for this transition is therefore essential. The PhD process is an opportunity to build your skillsets to help navigate this. *Note: Leaving the academy does not mean you cannot be academic.*

11.2 Finding Out What You Truly Enjoy

Whilst we can feel pressured (internally and externally) to just "knuckle down" and get our PhD work done, the benefits of extra-curricular work during the PhD process cannot be stressed enough. There will likely be a range of different ways you can contribute to the wider community and build skills during your PhD such as:

- Joining committees.
- Attending Learned Society Meetings.
- Connecting with peers and subject experts through social media.
- Writing for magazines.
- Equality, Diversity and Inclusion work.
- Joining (and even running) student societies.
- Reviewing papers.
- Running outreach events.

Of course, the balance of these in relation to doing your PhD research is important. You have a PhD to complete at the end of the day, so finding what balance works for you and not burning out is needed. This is often trial and error. Doing extra-curricular work can have huge benefits in terms of building contacts, as well as helping you figure out what work you enjoy, and what work you really do not. There is huge power in both.

One of the caveats around doing additional work is much of it is unpaid, and despite what some people say, "experience" and "exposure" really do not pay the bills. To this end, if this extra work is eating into self-care time, or means that combined with your PhD work you have little to no energy left, the extra-curricular work may have to take a back seat. In these situations, asking for time to do this work specifically during your PhD hours can be helpful. In the eventuality that something has to give, it is worth remembering that for most of this extra work you are volunteering your time, and asking for extensions or a hiatus, or even stepping away from the work entirely, is at your discretion. Another common issue is that Equality, Diversity and Inclusion (EDI) work often falls heavily on already underrepresented (historically marginalised) groups. This can be a heavy burden—not doing the work means that perhaps less people will be inspired to continue in academia, but doing the work means less time to do actual research, and as a member of a marginalised community, with the odds of success in academia already stacked against you, deciding on the best course of action can be extremely difficult. Further, EDI work despite its importance is often not given the same weighting as other academic work like publishing papers. This is a research culture issue. I cannot tell you what the "right" decision is for you on whether to invest your time in EDI initiatives. I can however tell you that whatever your decision, you have to do what is right for you and your career.

If you are experiencing significant pushback from your PhD Supervisor to not do "extra-curricular activities" it is worth noting that some funding bodies expect professional development opportunities to be included as part of your PhD training. Further, if doing a task is going to add to your CV and take a small amount of time, sometimes it is better to ask for forgiveness than permission.[3]

---

[3] It is worth noting that your PhD Supervisor will likely know how much time you need to put into your primary research, so it is important to listen to them, and most have your best interests at heart. If trying something new is important to you, explaining its value to your Supervisor might be the best approach.

11.3 Reframing Your Skillsets

Now, perhaps it is not traditional when talking about mental health to focus on the skills that you have learnt during your PhD and how translatable they are, but I think this is necessary based on my own experience transitioning from academia to industry [9]. If we feel as though we are pigeonholed into a particular career direction, or that we have not developed the skillsets we need to branch out of academia this can add stress and ultimately affect mental health. Worrying about "What comes next?" can also add significant stress. So what skills are you learning as you go through your PhD?

Learning to Learn…Fast One of the biggest and most translatable skills that you are learning during your PhD program is how to learn. Not only that, but how to process complex information, fast. This is a hugely valuable skill in academia, industry and beyond. It also means that if you decide to change research direction you know where to start—typically reading around a subject and not being afraid to ask questions.

Managing Large Projects Your PhD project is similar to running large research endeavours outside of academia. You are demonstrating the ability to time manage, plan ahead, and course-correct where necessary which are all hugely valuable skills.

Supporting Students The chances are that during your PhD program you are going to get the opportunity to support undergraduate research projects, and will frequently help PhD Students around you (particularly those just starting out). This is all people management and leadership skills and can be used as examples of such.

Managing Finances Your PhD may require you to order consumables, pay for conferences and purchase equipment. All of this requires some understanding of budgets, as well as searching for the best possible prices.

Collaboration and Connections Working as a team is a highly valued skill in all jobs, and shows that you can work creatively with a diverse team of people. Having a network of people you know within your field can also be beneficial not only to yourself but also to future employers.

Understanding Challenging Concepts You have demonstrated the ability to critically think and problem solve, as well as get to grips with challenging concepts. These skills are highly translatable to any work that comes next.

Communication Skills Writing and presenting on your research during your PhD demonstrates that you have built up confidence to present your work, as well as developed the ability to present complex information in a clear, easy to understand manner. *Note: You should be taught these during your PhD study. If not, you are within your rights to ask for support.*

Now, perhaps you are not getting experience of some of the skills I have listed here. It may be that there is no opportunity within your PhD position to explore some of these. But this also highlights the power of asking for opportunities too. For example, asking to manage a master's student project. Not only can this build confidence but lead to increased skillsets that make you highly competitive for your next role.

11.4 Transitioning from Your PhD

After completing your PhD, the next big challenge is managing the uncertainty of what comes next. Juggling searching for jobs and writing up can be very stressful. The first step in this process is to explore what you want to do in the first place. A good exercise is to think critically about what you want in each of the following areas to help determine your next steps:

Self What are your values? What parts of your work do you enjoy? What do you dislike?

Strengths What are you good at? What skills have you picked up during your PhD?

Networks Who can get you to where you want to go? How might they help you? Have you got a clear online profile (such as LinkedIn or a personal website) and is it up to date?

Opportunities What options are out there for someone with your skillset? If there is something you want to do, but you don't feel fully qualified, what experience do you need to get?

Want Do you want to move country? Would you rather stay living where you are?

Need Do you need a job immediately?

Understanding these questions can really help determine your next actions. For example, if you have to pay your rent/mortgage, getting a job doing anything to pay your bills to start with may be the only option. This will dictate the range of jobs you apply for and how much time is necessary to put in to applications.[4]

You may also feel overwhelmed balancing thesis writing and job applications at the same time. Prioritisation really comes into play here. Job posts are typically cyclical, with most job application windows being open for at least a week. This means that job applications can likely be limited to one or two days a week, allowing you to focus on your thesis for the rest of the time, without missing out on opportunities.

Many universities and professional bodies also run CV writing workshops to assist you in the job application process—take advantage of these. Further, if you have a mentor, a postdoc in your research group, or even your PhD Supervisor, they may be able to look over your CV and double check the content. If you are applying for varied job roles, it may also be worth making CVs tailored to the areas you are applying to, for example "Senior Scientist", "Lab Manager" "Research Assistant", where different key skills are highlighted, and the most suitable one can be used for applying to particular job roles, with minimal editing to speed up the application process.

11.5   Debunking the Myths

There are a range of myths that we might hear during the PhD process, which might put us off exploring work outside of the academy. It is important to address these as many of them are just that—myths [9].

Myth 1: There is no way to be creative outside of academia
We can be so concerned about having the academic freedoms to explore what we want that we can think that academia is the only place for us. Yet there are thousands of jobs outside of academia that rely on creativity and doing research.
Myth 2: Academia is more flexible for family life
Academic work can be flexible, particularly during school vacation time, providing time to look after children or do other caring responsibilities. This does not mean that it is not possible to achieve this outside of academia. Many companies operate with core hours, enabling flexible working. It is also important to remember that even though academia appears flexible there is a huge

---

[4] Personally, when looking for my next job, I wanted to stay in roughly the same location, so that limited my job search to a particular locale.

number of working hours that are often not written on the work contract but are often expected nonetheless.

Myth 3: Leaving academia is "selling your soul"

Going to work for industry can often be touted as "selling your soul" or giving in to capitalism in some way. There is no shame in wanting to have your skills valued, or earn more money. You must do what is right for you.

Myth 4: If you leave academia you cannot return

While it may be more difficult to return to academia if you leave, this is not necessarily the case. Many people return to study later in life. Further, some of the most sought after lecturers have industrial experience.

Myth 5: You are not an academic if you are not at a university

Often, being an "academic study" is associated with university settings, but the two are not exclusive to one another. You can be an academic inside and outside of the academy. Leaving the university setting does not take this away. Nor are research jobs exclusive to university settings (I say this to you as someone working in industry writing this academic book).

11.6   Should I Stay or Should I Go?

Deciding to pursue a career in academia is not something I can advise you on from here. It truly does depend on your unique situation. There is no right or wrong answer.

Sometimes we need to put ourselves first. Constantly up-ending your life to move to a new institution or new country every year due to the precarity of postdoctoral contracts may not be okay for you. This doesn't mean that you are not committed to research, just that your priorities are focused on your wellbeing. Whilst international moves can be exciting, the pressure to move country to build a competitive CV can be complicated, and might mean leaving your support network behind, which is essential for you to maintain good mental health. You may deem this worth it for your shot at your dream job in academia—the point is, it is your choice to make.

Further, continuing on to do a postdoctoral position in academia as it is the most convenient option for you, is more than okay, even if you have no intention of staying in academia long-term. Again, a range of skills you learn during postdoctoral work are translatable to jobs outside of the academy, so you are not just wasting time or delaying the inevitable by staying for a while. Sometimes having income and stability (even if it is only for a year or two) has to be a priority. And, maybe, just maybe, it might reignite your passion for academia.

In some cases, it is deemed that better work-life balance (and the better mental wellbeing that comes with it) is actually obtainable in industry/government jobs outside of academia. This of course depends heavily on the organisation and working culture they foster. During the time of writing this book, the SARS-CoV-2 pandemic is ongoing, and what has been termed the "great resignation", with university staff leaving academia, is happening for exactly this reason, with the pandemic adding strain onto an already strained system [10, 11].

Finally, it is also worth mentioning that "success" in academia does not equate to professorship. There are many jobs within academic settings, whether it is being a teaching fellow, a research fellow, being research adjacent, or a job in professional services. You do not need to be a professor to be happy and do research. Finally, if you are still absolutely sold on the idea of being a professor one day and it is a life-long dream of yours, know it is absolutely possible.

ADVOCATING FOR BETTER: How Can Career Uncertainty Be Improved for PhD Students?

Determining the next steps after PhD study can be overwhelming, particularly if a PhD student is having to juggle writing up their thesis as well as searching for a job. It is therefore important that universities prepare PhD students for the big "What's next?". In my opinion, this can be done by:

1. **Building in professional development**—Providing dedicated time for professional development per week/month, ensuring that PhD students are developing transferrable skills.
2. **Paint a realistic picture of the academic job market**—Being honest with PhD students about the competitive nature of academia and the lack of academic jobs is an important conversation, as this may not have been considered.
3. **Feature role models**—Seeing alternative jobs that are available as well as the individuals doing them can be incredibly powerful as both a motivator, and simply putting a spotlight on career options that may not have previously been considered.
4. **Consider the inclusion of a "extra-curricular" thesis chapter**—More recently there has been a push at some institutions to enable one thesis chapter to be about extra-curricular work done during PhD study and I hope to see this as a practise adopted in other universities too. This is hugely beneficial as it enables students to give back to their research community as well as develop new skills.
5. **Consider emergency funds**—Applying for a job during the write-up phase of a PhD if there are concerns over paying bills and rent is incredibly stressful. If possible funding should be available to ensure that PhD students do not have to worry about writing up with no income.

References

1. HESA (2022) Where do HE students come from? HESA, Cheltenham, UK
2. HESA (2021) Higher education staff statistics: UK, 2019/20. HESA, Cheltenham, UK
3. HESA (2022) Who's studying in HE? HESA, Cheltenham
4. Baker S (2021) Rapid rise in professors aged over 65 sparks opportunities debate. Times Higher Education
5. Woolston C (2019) PhDs: the tortuous truth. Nature 575(7782):403–407
6. Limas JC, Corcoran LC, Baker AN, Cartaya AE, Ayres ZJ (2022) The impact of research culture on mental health & diversity in STEM. Chemistry 28(9):e202102957
7. The Royal Society (2010) The scientific century - securing our future prosperity. The Royal Society, London, UK
8. Human Indicators Project (2021) State of the humanities 2021: workforce and beyond. AAAS, Cambridge, MA
9. Kelsky K (2015) The professor is in: the essential guide to turning your Ph.D. into a job. Crown, New York
10. Heffernan TA, Heffernan A (2019) The academic exodus: the role of institutional support in academics leaving universities and the academy. Prof Dev Educ 45(1):102–113
11. Gewin V (2022) Has the 'great resignation' hit academia? https://www.nature.com/articles/d41586-022-01512-6. Accessed 21 Jun 2022

Part IV

Seeking Help

12

Thriving, Not Just Surviving

As I stated at the start of this book, I am not a psychologist, nor am I trained in mental health support. To this end, I cannot provide medical guidance in this chapter. Instead, what follows is as starting point on how you might seek help for mental illness, as well as a list of resources I wish I had known about, that have helped myself and others throughout their own mental health journeys. I encourage you to explore other resources out there to figure out what might work best for you. Simply put: this is just a starting point on your journey to mental health management.[1]

To understand how to best look after your mental health during a PhD program, I see many parallels between seeking help and putting together a research proposal. For both there are three main elements: identifying the (research) problem set, sharing the hypothesis with others, and seeking external assistance from others to achieve your (research) goal.

Of course, it is incredibly easy to outline the research proposal process in these simple steps, but much, much, harder to put it into practice. The same is true for seeking mental health support. But it absolutely can be done—let's explore how.

(Trigger Warnings: suicidal ideation, depression)

---

[1] Personally I much prefer "mental health management" to "recovery" as in my own experience I have learned that my mental illness(es) are chronic, thus I likely will never "recover" from them, but to function well I certainly have had to learn to manage them.

Z. J. Ayres, *Managing your Mental Health during your PhD*,
https://doi.org/10.1007/978-3-031-14194-2_12

12.1   Identifying the Problem Set

Perhaps the biggest challenge those of us with mental illness can face is acknowledging that we need help for our mental health in the first place. A bigger challenge still, we have to accept that we **deserve** help. This can be particularly difficult when our self-worth is at its lowest, and we are struggling to see ourselves the way that those that love us see us—trust me I know this feeling all too well. And yet, everyone is worthy of help. We do not "earn" our right to live, or right to thrive, it is inherent. You deserve help just as much as anyone else.

Now, even though I have said this, you may not feel ready to reach out for help, because speaking it out loud means accepting that you are struggling. You also may be afraid of what others might think of you. These are all normal feelings, compounded by the societal stigma around mental illness. I am here to tell you that help is out here for when you are ready, whether it is today, tomorrow or in three months' time. There are people, whether they are medical professionals or friends and family that care about your wellbeing [1].

We can also be incredibly good at minimising our concerns, looking at others around us and thinking "they have it worse" and concluding that we don't actually need help ourselves. This is a false dichotomy. It is not "one or the other". Everyone deserves help, and whilst there may be a huge range in mental health experiences from person to person, suffering is not a competition. We can also have a tendency to think that we must have been experiencing mental illness for a prolonged period before seeking help. In reality, for a diagnosis, a change in mood can have been happening for as little as 2 weeks, and does not have to be constant (simply more days struggling than not) [2]. Further, the onset of mental illness can be described as "a change from or marked exaggeration of prior and normal state of functioning", which means that however you are feeling, if it is different from *your* normal, it may be time to seek help [2].

Task

In Chap. 2 we discussed "recognising the signs" of mental illness. I encourage you to go back and look at this list, and reflect on about how you are feeling. Does even one of these descriptors describe your experience? If so, it might be time to consider seeking some support.

Further, something I wish had learnt much earlier is that "functioning" does not mean fine. As intelligent individuals, to the outside world we may seem well put together and that we are "managing just fine", but if we are like a swan on water, looking elegant on the surface, but underneath paddling hard, struggling to stay afloat, we absolutely need to seek help. There is only so long that that façade will stand before it comes crumbling down.

12.2   Sharing the Hypothesis with Others

The next step in the process of managing your mental health is reaching out for support from those around you. If other people do not know you are struggling it is impossible for them to provide help and appropriate accommodations.

12.3   Conversation Starters

It can sometimes be difficult to know where to start when talking to someone about your mental health and asking for help, so here are some conversation starters to help you articulate how you might be feeling, as detailed in Boynton (2020) [1]:

- I have been feeling low for the last few weeks and I…
- I am struggling with my mental health…
- I need help with…
- I feel anxious about….
- I am not sure quite how to describe how I am feeling but…
- I am worried that you think I am disengaged but I have been really finding managing my mental health hard…
- I need to take a break…
- I feel like…
- I am burned out and…
- I am not okay right now…
- Please can we go for a coffee as I need to speak with you about…

If you are finding speaking to someone in person daunting, it is worth remembering that there are a range of different ways to communicate, from email, to through text, or social media. If you are struggling and don't know who to turn to, social media provides a good conduit to get support and guidance, and can provide anonymity if you do not feel like sharing with people you know to start with.

12.4   Finding a Support Network

Navigating your PhD alone can be a lonely journey. Finding people to share the experience with can make all the difference. There are a range of people based on your university campus and beyond that are here to help [1]. Here are just a few:

University Support University campuses have a range of mental health support available for PhD students. This typically includes student support services, disability support, counselling services and a chaplaincy. These resources are there for you to access. Most universities also have mental health support lines you can call as a listening service.

Your Cohort There is incredible power in connecting with other members of your cohort, as many of you will be experiencing similar issues, and if we think back to the statistics at the start of the book, approximately 1 in 2 PhD students will experience some form of mood disorder during their PhD. This means there is a high probability of finding some colleagues that you can relate to, and by connecting you can support each other. *Tip: Creating study groups, or organising social events may be a way to connect.*

Connecting with Others University clubs and societies provide a way to connect with others on your campus. If you are an international student, there may be specific societies to find people from your home country to connect with. This can help with culture shock and navigating a new country.

Ombudsman Your campus may have an Ombudsman who is an independent person that can help you navigate a complaints procedure if you have been unfairly treated by your university.

Union Most PhD students are classed as staff, and this means that you are entitled to join a union. Your union representative can help you know your rights if you find yourself in a tricky situation. It's not always know that as a PhD student you may be able to join at a reduced rate, or in some cases membership is free.

Disability Office As a PhD student, there are likely a range of different accommodations available to you to help you with your mental health, as well as managing other disabilities. By understanding what is available to you, this may help to alleviate significant strain. Your student disability office (or similar) on campus should be able to point you in the direction of useful resources.

12.5 Online Communities

It may not be news for you—I am an avid fan of social media, particularly Twitter. Sometimes it can be difficult to find people that understand our mental illnesses at our own institutions, but by connecting with the wider research community we can make connections with people that can truly appreciate what we are going through. There are a range of communities online, as well as hashtags (some useful ones listed below, accurate as of Summer 2022) where you can get involved in the conversation, or simply observe learnings from the community:

#NEISVoid—Standing for "No End In Sight" this is a space for those with chronic illness to discuss navigating challenges as well as successes.
#BlackInTheIvory—Discussions of racism within the academy.
#AcademicMentalHealth—General discussions on mental health issues and stories from people within academia at all career stages.
#PhDChat—General discussions on PhD life, covering the highs and the lows.
#AcademicChatter, #AcademicTwitter—Discussions from academics at all career stages in in the academy exploring daily life, successes, and struggles.
#ActuallyAutistic—Accounts from the autistic community.
#ADHD—Discussions about navigating life with Attention Deficit Hyperactivity Disorder.
#DisInHigherEd—A community discussing navigating higher education with disability.
#MeToo—A space for discussions around sexual harassment.

12.6   Speaking About Your Mental Health with Your PhD Supervisor

It can feel like a daunting task to discuss your mental health with your PhD Supervisor, and yet the majority of PhD Supervisors want to see their PhD Students succeed. Here is the thing: Your PhD Supervisor cannot help if they do not know there is an issue. If you are struggling, your supervisor may have noticed a change in your behaviour, and may bring it up themselves. If you do not know how to broach the topic, consider sending an email first outlining what you wish to discuss [3]. Consider using the "conversation starters" as a way to start dialogue around your mental health with your PhD Supervisor.

In some instances your PhD Supervisor might not know what support is out there for you (even though they should). It is well within your right to ask them to find out more information for you. I also want to mention that it is absolutely okay to not disclose to your PhD Supervisor too, if you do not feel safe to do so.

12.7   Lack of Understanding

When you open up to someone about how you are feeling and do not get the response you hoped for it can be hurtful. In some cases, those we care about may carry stigma around mental health concerns themselves or be in denial because they did not realise you were struggling. We may even hear unhelpful phrases like "Oh well we are all depressed right now" or "Pull yourself together".

Sometimes even those around us who truly care and want to help and provide support can get it wrong, as they do not understand what you are going through, as they have never experienced mental illness themselves. Although disheartening, I suggest speaking to someone else about your mental health concerns, as there will be people that *do* understand around you, be it a colleague or a medical professional. In short: please do not let one bad interaction put you off seeking help.

12.8   Seeking External Assistance to Achieve Your Goal

Sometimes, just like we often have to do to improve research outcomes, you may have to seek external help for your mental health. In this case, instead of a collaborator, we look to medical professionals for guidance. There is no shame in needing support to get well again.

Most PhD programs in high income countries have some sort of medical care built in as standard for being on a PhD program. This may be access to medical care as well as access to short-term therapy. In LMICs, there may be no medical/financial support.[2]

It is important to remember that mental health stigma and bias can be present within the medical community too. If you think there is something wrong with how you are feeling, there is no-one who is more of an expert in that than you. It is more than reasonable to seek a second (or even third) opinion from a medical professional. For most interactions though, medical professionals are there to help you, and want you to feel well again. Ringing your local doctor or General Practitioner and booking an appointment to discuss how you are feeling is the first step in seeking this help. *Tip: If you are worrying about what you are going to say, write the main points you want to communicate down before you ring your doctor.*

There is also much stigma associated with seeking medical help, as well as common misnomers. I want to challenge a few of these here [4]:

Myth 1: Medication is for the weak
Just like if you were experiencing hypertension, or diabetes, medication is often needed to manage mental illness. This is not a weakness, it is an illness.

Myth 2: Only a formal diagnosis matters
Whilst a formal diagnosis may give you access to medications and accommodations to help, self-diagnosis is absolutely valid. In order to seek a formal diagnosis, first we have to suspect that we might have a condition in the first place. Further, formal diagnosis can be expensive, and thus not a tangible option for some.

Myth 3: Therapy is a last resort [5]
Representation of therapy in pop-culture often seems to indicate that it is a last resort for mental health management. In reality it is beneficial not just at crisis point but throughout our lives to help us understand the world around us and why we feel the way we do.

Myth 4: Medication will completely change your personality
It is only by trying medication that you can really see the effect it may have, but there is a long-standing myth that taking medication will change you into an entirely different person, and mean you can no longer be you. This is quite simply not the case.

Myth 5: The side effects are awful
Mental health medication has advanced significantly, and with any medication, your progress will be monitored carefully by your medical professional.

---

[2] This is a huge failing at the institutional level, and if you are subjected to this, I am so sorry. Affordable medical support and access is a basic human right.

If you experience any side effects that you are unhappy with this can all be fed back to your medical advisor, and alternatives can be found. In some cases side effects can cause issues,[3] but medication for mental illness is used regularly, to great effect, by people all around the world. There are many alternatives to investigate if the first medication you try doesn't work well for you.

12.9   If You Are at Crisis Point

Being at crisis point means feeling like you are at breaking point, and need assistance urgently. You may be [1]:

- Suicidal, including experiencing suicidal ideation.
- Self-harming.
- Feeling anxious.
- Experiencing panic attacks, or PTSD flashbacks.
- Feeling high (experiencing hypomania).
- Feeling paranoid.
- Hearing voices (experiencing psychosis).

In this instance, urgent care is needed. There are range of options available to you, from speaking to friends and family, calling (or texting) your local country mental health charity helplines, as well as going directly to your local hospital for help.

If you are worried about reaching crisis point, it may be valuable to put together your own "Safety Plan", where pre-emptively you write down answers to questions, including why you want to live, where to get help, and how to make the environment you are in safer for yourself when experiencing suicidal thoughts [1, 6]. Several links to online Safety Plans, including one by the UK mental health charity Samaritans are detailed in the additional resources weblink at the back of the book.

---

[3] I myself occasionally experience night sweats on my fluoxetine (Prozac) tablets but I deemed this a small price to pay for improved mood.

12.10   The Elephant in the Room

I now want to take a moment to talk about the elephant in the room—quitting your PhD. Nothing, and I mean absolutely nothing, is worth your peace of mind. Certainly not a doctorate. So whilst many of you will "push through", perseverance has a limit. If you find yourself in a toxic environment where your mental health is being negatively impacted (so much so that you have given up hope), you can and must leave your PhD program. There is no shame in this. You deserve better than that. It is more than okay to walk away from a situation that is not built for you to succeed. Sometimes quitting a PhD program is the biggest act of self-care we can do.

We can also delay leaving due to the fear of what friends and family might think, yet those who love you will understand if you explain your situation to them. You may also fear your next steps and how best to explain to a future employer or your next PhD Supervisor about your decision to leave, but know that you are highly employable and the skills you have learnt during your PhD stint (however short) bring huge value. There is also often the option to gain a master's degree instead of a PhD if you are part way through, which again is highly valued.

There is often much negativity around the word "quit", but I prefer to think about quitting using the Middle English etymology route, which means to be "set free". It is okay to leave if you need to.

12.11   Leading the Change

Not everyone is in a position to talk openly about mental health, particularly in a public setting. This is more than okay—you owe your mental health journey to no-one. There may be some of you though, that look at the current support available at your university for PhD students and note that it is lacking. This might inspire you to drive for change within your own department. At the end of each chapter, there have been some "Advocating for Better" suggestions for you to utilise to drive for change in your institutions if you so wish. Expanding on how we implement these changes needs much more work as a research community, and is a great place to start discussions.

From my own experience of advocating for change when it comes to academic mental health, I wanted to share some of my learnings with you:

Lead with Data To make change, a convincing argument is needed. This involves collecting evidence of mental health concerns in regards to PhD students. Thankfully this book (see Chap. 3) and many other resources are out there to help. If your department want more localised data, and there isn't any, a survey is a good place to start. Caution must be practiced though—a survey if well-meant, but poorly designed, may not collect useful information.

Don't Make It "Us vs. Them" It's easy to raise a pitchfork and tell senior management that they need to do better, but this is very unlikely to get results. It is important to remember that this lack of mental health provision is systemic, not personal, and that only by students and staff working together can real change be brought about.

Find Allies Creating change is much easier if the burden is shared. Find allies around you that are also invested in improving mental health support at your university. This is especially important if you struggle with your own mental health from time to time, so that you can step back when you need space and time to look after yourself.

Expect Some Resistance When proposing changes, it is often the case we might hear "Well this is how it has always been done" or "We don't have budget for that". This can make making improvements an uphill struggle. *Tip: Starting small can still propagate change, like hosting a student discussion to talk about mental health support that is available.*

Do Not Be Disheartened Change takes time, and in academia change can be glacial. This doesn't mean that advocacy work isn't helping others. It's often the case that you may not get positive feedback for the work you are doing as it takes a lot of energy for individuals to come forward.

The Most Important Thing Is You Sometimes advocacy work can take its toll. It is okay to step back from it for a while, and come back to it when you are able. There should be no guilt attached to prioritising you and your wellbeing.

12.12   Not Just Surviving

My honest hope is that one day there will be no need for this book, or at the very least the systemic issues section will be redundant. There should be no need for a PhD "Survival Guide" in the first place. It should not be difficult to navigate higher education. Everyone has a right to further education, and everyone intrinsically brings value.

Throughout this book, I have explored the PhD experience. In the first section, we focused on what you can do as an individual to help bolster your resilience and work towards a more informed, positive mindset when it comes to your PhD studies. This was not included to patronise, or tell you what you already know, but as a reminder that there are parts of our PhD life in our control that when well managed can help us on our PhD journey. This includes getting your "foundations" right when it comes to self-care, with the knowledge that investing in you means you are more likely to be able to manage in the lower, lonelier moments of your PhD. This means an investment in self-care, ensuring that you are eating well, getting enough sleep, and exercising (where possible). It is also important to realise that if you do not have access to these, be it due to financial difficulties or due to chronic illness etc., this is not your fault. It just means that alternative support systems may be even more important for you in order to succeed. Building your mental health "toolkit" is an essential investment in you.

We also explored that sometimes the biggest barrier we might encounter on our PhD journey is ourselves: the negative self-talk that accompanies the impostor phenomenon; the self-imposed guilt we often feel for not working constantly; the letting go of all our self-care in the pursuit of a deadline and the punishing ourselves for not being as "productive as we should have been". Recognising these patterns, calling out our inner voice, and questioning if we would say the same things to a friend can be a good start in managing our own thoughts. This may require you to explore resources available to you, including project and time management tools, calibrating your expectations by finding someone to mentor you through the PhD process, and taking regular (much deserved) breaks away from research to come back refreshed.

I have also explored systemic issues that may affect you as a PhD student as you go through your studies. This is not a damning indictment of one or two universities, but a reflection on academia as a whole. One of the most important take-aways from this book, is that mental health support and provision is not simply an individual responsibility, but that of the university we are studying for our PhD at. The environment we find ourselves in can have huge impact on whether we can succeed. To assist in this, in the third section of this book, we explored "environmental stressors" detailing some of the systemic challenges you might face.

I also want to leave you with some final take-home thoughts that I carry with me that stemmed from my own PhD and mental illness experience, that I wish I had known at the times when I was struggling. I hope they will benefit you too:

We Are Not Research Machines We have feelings, emotions. We might find we end up crying in our PhD Supervisor's office more than once. That doesn't make us unprofessional—it simply makes us human. And it is this human element that brings curiosity and caring for the world around us: the very reason we go into research in the first place.

If It Was Easy It Would Already Be Done With PhD research you are standing on the shoulders of giants, trying to discover something new, understand it, then put it out in the world. This is no small feat. It is going to be hard to make new discoveries and piece all that information together—it is part of the process. It will take time, study, and luck to find something new, and you may end up discovering something entirely unrelated to your initial studies. The finish line will not be visible for quite some time.

You Have Already Proven Your Capability It is easy to forget, we actually have the skills to succeed during a PhD already from our previous experiences. This is why to do a PhD in the first place there is a range of acceptance criteria. You qualified for your PhD position, not through some kind of fluke (you are not an impostor), and you deserve your PhD position.

Suffering Is Not a Standard When we talk about a PhD being difficult, this should refer to the research being challenging, not experiencing bullying behaviour or being told to fend for yourself with little to no support. There is no "rite of passage" for entry into a PhD program, nor do you have to prove yourself. Research is hard enough without someone trying to make it even more difficult for you.

Comparison Is the Thief of Joy No one person's journey (be it their research career or their background) is the same. Thus, it is not valid to compare yourself with those around you.

Luck and Privilege Is the Unmentioned Success Factor You can try and try to succeed at your research, but that doesn't necessarily mean that you will get the outcome you were looking for. Whilst "everyone has the same 24 hours in a day" not everyone has the same luck, project or privilege. Academia is not a meritocracy.

You and Your Wellbeing Has to Be the Priority When managing a mental illness and doing a PhD program, you will likely have to set boundaries to protect your mental health. Otherwise the culture of overwork may lead to burnout. Do not take your physical or mental health for granted—nothing is worth the expense of them.

Walking Away Is Okay If you find yourself in a toxic, oppressive working environment, that is not your fault. You have every right to look after yourself and walk away, re-evaluate your options and try something new. You have not failed, academia has failed *you*.

There Is a Whole Host of Systemic Issues Within the Academy Whilst not often mentioned, the academy itself is flawed. There are many barriers to success that individuals might face, particularly from historically marginalised groups. These issues are systemic, and should not happen, but they do. It is important to remember that if you are struggling, it might be them not you.

Academia Needs You Perhaps one day, if you beat the odds and become a professor (and I truly hope for you that if you want it you make it), you'll reflect back and realise that the power is yours to make a difference from top-down. True leadership intersects heavily with compassion, and those of us living with mental illness often have compassion in spades. To improve academia, academia needs more disabled academics in leadership roles.

For those of you struggling right now, know mental illness does not define our capability, or our potential. We can claim it as a descriptor for ourselves, or never tell a soul. It is our choice. But either way, we should celebrate that our experience with mental illness(es) brings a unique perspective that is vital for research, and for improving the world around us for the better.

There may be days where life is an uphill struggle; where the challenge of the day is not world-leading research, but simply getting out of bed. On others, the finish line may seem so out of sight that it appears impossible to reach. On those days I ask you to remind yourself that you deserve your PhD position and hang on to the fact that tomorrow always has the potential to be better.

On other days—on the rare days where research works—revel in it. Share your joy with others. Celebrate the little wins, as well as the big ones, and try to hold on to that feeling for as long as you can.

Finally, if you do find yourself in the dark, lonely place I found myself in during my PhD, I say this to you now: You are so much more than your PhD. Your worth is not measured by your academic achievements. You are deserving of help, and there is help out here for you when you are ready.

One thing I can tell you categorically: you are absolutely *not alone*. And although you might not be able to see it yet, somewhere, in the not so distant future, be it within academia, or finding your worth elsewhere, there is a version of you that is not just surviving, but thriving.

References

1. Boynton P (2020) Being well in academia: Ways to Feel Stronger, Safer and More Connected. Routledge, Abingdon
2. World Health Organisation (1992) Classification of mental and behavioural disorders. WHO, Geneva
3. Saló-Salgado L, Acocella A, Arzuaga García I, El Mousadik S, Zvinavashe A (2021) Managing up: how to communicate effectively with your PhD adviser. https://www.nature.com/articles/d41586-021-03703-z. Accessed 15 Feb 2022
4. Serani D (2021) 6 Antidepressant medication myths. https://www.psychologytoday.com/gb/blog/two-takes-depression/202009/6-antidepressant-medication-myths. Accessed 21 Jun 2022
5. VanDerBill B (2021) 7 Myths and facts about psychotherapy. https://psychcentral.com/health/myths-about-therapy. Accessed 21 Jun 2022
6. Samaritans (2022) Supporting someone with suicidal thoughts. https://www.samaritans.org/how-we-can-help/if-youre-worried-about-someone-else/supporting-someone-suicidal-thoughts/creating-safety-plan/. Accessed 15 Feb 2022

Resources

When writing this book I originally was going to create a resources section at the back of the book, but the more I thought about it, the more I realised that there are so many good resources out there that are constantly evolving, that I simply would not be able to cover them all and do a reasonable job simply writing them in the book. Instead I have created the webpage:

www.zjayres.com/phdresources

which has an up to date list of resources available to you, with submissions from individuals from around the world going through a similar experience to you. If you know of a resource that other PhD students may benefit from that is not on the list, please do get in touch! This will be an ever evolving webpage, curated by me, informed by the PhD community.

CPSIA information can be obtained
at www.ICGtesting.com
Printed in the USA
LVHW080531101022
730300LV00001B/2